CLINICAL WRITING
FOR
HEALTH PROFESSIONALS

Alice M. Robinson, R.N., M.S.
and
Lucille E. Notter, R.N., Ed.D.

Robert J. Brady Co., Bowie, Md.
A Prentice-Hall Publishing
and
Communications Company

Executive Producer: Richard A. Weimer
Production Editor: Paula K. Aldrich
Art Director: Donald E. Sellers

Clinical writing for health professionals.

Library of Congress Cataloging in Publication Data

Robinson, Alice M.
  Clinical writing for health professionals

  Includes bibliographies and index.
  1. Medical writing. I. Notter, Lucille E.
II. Title. [DNLM: 1. Writing. WZ 345 R658c]
R119.R62   808:06661021   81-3821
ISBN 0-87619-893-0   AACR2

Prentice-Hall International, Inc., London
Prentice-Hall of Australia, Pty., Ltd., Sydney
Prentice-Hall of India Private Limited, New Delhi
Prentice-Hall of Japan, Inc., Tokyo
Prentice-Hall of Southeast Asia Pte. Ltd., Singapore
Whitehall Books, Limited, Petone, New Zealand

Printed in the United States of America

82 83 84 85 86 87 88 89 90 91 92   10 9 8 7 6 5 4 3 2 1

CONTENTS

Preface

PART ONE

PREFACE

I published my first article in the late 1940's. It was the first manuscript I had ever submitted and was a runner-up in a writer's contest conducted by the successful, then pocket-sized *RN Magazine*. Alice Clarke, the editor of *RN* at the time, decided that since it presented a new concept in psychiatric nursing, she would publish it, even though it wasn't a contest winner.

It was easier to get published in those days because not many health professionals were writing, and the age of "publish or perish" in academia had not yet taken hold. That professional success cliché (publish or perish) is back with us in the 80s, and it still embarks professionals on the lecture and publishing tours, and it sets them up for bigger and better professional job opportunities.

The professional who wants to publish today shouldn't be an amateur because the competition is getting keen and, even though the editors of professional journals are happy to "work over" a poorly written article that has a new, sound idea, the working over may eliminate any originality or personal style of the author. It is much better for the aspiring writer to learn the basic skills of clinical professional writing and become known not only for his expertise, but for a fresh, new style that sets him apart as a recognized writer among his peers.

This little book is actually the result of a number of inquiries I have received about the clinical professional writing course I conduct as director of Specialized Consultants in Nursing. Following national publicity in the better known nursing journals, I began to receive letters from individuals who wanted to participate in "the next writing workshop."

Because the writing course is both difficult to take and difficult ot teach, it is limited to a small number of students, which didn't begin to answer the requests from all over the country.

When the Robert J. Brady Company approached me to "exchange ideas" and see if I was ready to write another book, I proposed a clinical professional writing text to help answer the need for not only launching people into publishing, but, more important, helping them turn out a well written communication, whether interdepartmental memorandum, business letter, resume, article or book.

I am indebted to Dr. Lucille Notter, who wrote the valuable Part Two of the book, for her infinite patience with my procrastination, and for the contribution she has made to this effort. Undoubtedly, she is the best person to do so.

Many other people have been supportive and helpful in this venture, but I am particularly indebted to Alice R. Clarke, now editor and publisher of Nursing Publications, Inc., Fanny Siegel, director, Program of Continuing Education, Teachers College Columbia University, and my cousin, Lillian Adams, who typed the manuscript. I am also deeply appreciative of the continued prompting and support of Richard Weimer of the Robert J. Brady Company.

Alice M. Robinson, R.N., M.S.

PART ONE

CHAPTER 1: Improving Written Communications

People engaged in the health care professions—nurses, physicians, social workers, researchers, graduate students, and so on—need to learn to communicate, *in writing,* in an effective, meaningful way. There is a great demand for help in this area, and with the increasing number of health care journals entering the publishing arena, there is also tremendous competition for publishable manuscripts.

There are many hurdles on the road to publication and even the experienced author trips over more than a few before he sees his article in print. More often than not, the road is also a long one—and can be discouraging to the expert as well as the neophyte. Unless you are a genius like F. Scott Fitzgerald or Agatha Christie, you'll wait a long time, and wade through some disheartening rejection slips before you make the grade.

Although the rules of style, as set forth in other texts, are not infallible, it is essential that a serious writer learn them almost to the point that they become second nature to him. In other words, there are times when, for clarity or simplicity, or just because it reads better, a rule can be altered. In general, it is better to stick by the wise dictums of those who, after long experience, have written them down for us.

To quote from the most widely used book of style, "It is an old observation that the best writers sometimes disregard the rules of rhetoric. When they do so, however, the reader will usually find in the sentence some compensating merit, attained at the cost of the violation."*

---

*Strunk, William, Jr., and White, E. B. *The Elements of Style.* Second ed., 1972, The Macmillan Co., New York City.

Notes on Patients

Health care professionals and the facilities they work in are well known for their inadequate and sometimes even ludicrous communications or systems of communication. The use of computers in larger institutions is helping some to overcome outright confusion, but they are prohibitively expensive for many facilities, so the misspelled, misstated, and misunderstood messages will be with us for a while.

Physicians' notes have come to be known as nontranslatable, not so much because of what they say as the fact that many physicians have perfected the art of indecipherable handwriting even before they leave medical school. Abbreviations, acronyms, and symbols in medicine are also a part of the problem, as shown by the following:

> A doctor read the day nurse's brief report: "Pt. c/o SOB most of the day." He wrote underneath: "Probably in CHF. Prognosis? GOK." And then, in parentheses, he jotted down: "In case you're not up on that, it means, 'God only knows.'"*

That anecdote shows us that some nurses are no less guilty. Nurses have been traditionally taught to write legibly but also to say nothing that might incriminate them—and that translates to "nothing!" A sample of the *traditional* nurses' notes over 24 hours goes like this:

> 8 A.M. — 4 P.M. Morning care given
> Patient OOB
> Still not eating. 1,000 cc D/W
> started I.V. Running well.

---

*Reprinted from *RN Magazine,* Jan., 1975. Copyright © 1975 by Medical Economics Co., Oradell, NJ 07649. All rights reserved.

4 P.M. — 12 Mn. I.V. disc. c̄ 750cc absorbed
                 Dr. visited
                 Soup 60cc, tea 90cc
                 Husband visited
12 Mn. — 8 A.M. Slept well
                 OOB to bathroom

Social workers have been better at writing their client histories and summarizing at discharge, and graduate students have had to write clearly; but, in turn, they have had journalism and English professors available to help them.

Fortunately, things are changing for the better in all the health disciplines. The impetus has come largely from more demanding education programs and from the promulgation of intensive and coronary care units where the foregoing sample of nurses' notes couldn't be tolerated. By comparison, the following is a nursing observation written on an actual patient in a neurosurgical intensive care unit:

12/3/79
9:50 A.M.   Seen by MD. ICP line flushed.
            ICP at 26.
10:00 A.M. N/S perl (sm) c̄ hg. RVE decorticate
            RVE decerebrate LE— pain, resp. to
            pain at times opens eyes
            ICP monitor recalibration by res-
            piratory therapy. Line flushed by MD.
            ICP fluctuating between 20-30 at times
            30-40. MD aware. Gastric pk. 65.
            Slight coffee ground material.

                M.M. _____ R.N.

Sophisticated, to be sure; intelligible and informative to those persons who work in neurosurgical ICUs but few others would understand it.

Any observation written by a health professional is a potentially legal communication, and thus, a potentially

3

lethal communication. More and more malpractice suits are being brought against not just physicians, but nurses, medical librarians, administrators, and others. Because these suits are occurring more frequently, lawyers request total patients' records and parts of patients' records, and they have learned what to look for. Even an unintentional error, no matter how much innocence is protested by the writer, can turn a jury's or judge's verdict around.

It is sad but true that the average person doesn't seem to be aware of some of the most important rules that govern the writing of "potentially lethal" documents.

Notices and Memorandums

Notices are usually informal, and can't do much damage, but a carelessly written notice may lose its impact. Recently I was teaching a course in a midwest hospital, and as we were walking through a basement corridor on the way to the cafeteria, we stopped to read this notice:

ALL PERSONNEL

Please don't hang your cats in the hall.
Put them in your lockers.
Housekeeping

The vision brought up by that one was amazing enough not to be taken seriously. There were still *coats* hanging in the hall.

Memorandums are usually written only about important matters (or should be saved for those), and they *can* be used as legal evidence. One of the exercises I give my writing course participants is to write a memorandum, usually on the basis of a controversial slide I show them.

Here is the controversial slide:

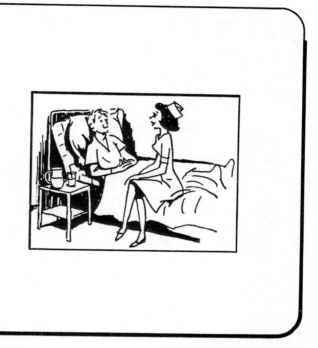

And here is a sample of a careless memo about it:

To: Head Nurse
From: Evening staff nurse
Last night I saw P.K.N. lounging on Peter's bed having a pretty intimate conversation with him. I think this was very unprofessional behavior and you should counsel her as soon as possible.

Again, the flaws are obvious—"Evening staff nurse" is misrepresenting the incident with her subjective terms "lounging" and "a pretty intimate conversation"; the mysterious staff nurse is also telling the head nurse how—and when—to handle the situation.

The flaws we need to be concerned about are not as obvious to the uninitiated. Most important, there is not a sign of a date or specific time in this memo; second, it is not directed to a person, just a title; nor do we know who wrote it or who "Peter" is. All of these faults would render it useless as an official document of any kind.

Here is a sample of a correctly written memo about an important unit meeting:

May 5, 1979

To: All personnel on Brown Unit
From: Paul S. Green, M.D.
Subject: Charting revision
The medical records committee has been reviewing the charting system on the Brown Unit because there have been some serious charting discrepancies made in the area of recording the giving of medications. There will be a meeting of all Unit personnel who regularly write on patients' charts, at 2 P.M., Wednesday, May 9, Unit conference room. Please try to be there.

If you follow these simple rules when writing memorandums, your messages will be effective:

1. Be sure month, day, year, and if necessary, the hour, are clear.
2. When possible, direct the memo to a specific name and title.
3. Give your name and title as the person writing the memo. Initial or sign your name.
4. Avoid being subjective—*"state the facts."*
5. Check for clarity and spelling.

Here's another situation to try writing a memo on:

An older man, part-time social worker, appears later and later on the mornings he is assigned to the unit. Following his sessions with them, the patients he is seeing appear somewhat upset. The unit secretary reports to you, confidentially, that she has smelled liquor on his breath on more than one occasion.

Who would you direct your memo to? Would you mention the unit secretary's comments? Would you include information about patients' reactions? Would you suggest a solution? If so, what?

Letters

Some people are born letter writers—whether they are writing personal or business letters. But they aren't in the majority, and there are some rules that can help you write more effective letters.

Several of the principles that govern memo writing also apply to letter writing; i.e., always give the date, address it to the person and title, avoid subjectivity, highlight the purpose of the letter, check your spelling and the clarity of your message.

If you know the person at all, a certain degree of informality is quite permissible. In this day and age—especially in the business world—people are not averse to first names. But—let the other person use *your* first name first.

You can sign a business letter in other ways than the traditional "Sincerely," "Respectfully," "Cordially," and so on. "Best personal regards," "Warm regards," or, if appropriate, "Happy Holidays," are all acceptable to most colleagues or professional friends.

Try to avoid being trite or commonplace. Try to be refreshing—but not at the expense of coming off as flippant. Business letters can be interesting, but it takes skill. And skill takes practice. There is nothing wrong with rewriting or revising a business letter several times before you send out the final version. It is wise, incidentally, to avoid such obviously conjured up phrases as, "This writer believes," or "Your attention to the above matter," or "Thanking you in advance for your attention to this matter."

Query letters regarding manuscripts to be submitted for publication will be dealt with later.

Biographical Data

Putting together one's professional biographical data, or resumé, should be a very careful process. The professional resumé is submitted for a number of purposes: seeking a new position; telling an editor (and eventually your readers) who and what you are and what you've done; preparing to enter an academic program; giving the person who's introducing you as a speaker some idea of how to tell the audience why you are there; and so forth.

The most common misconception resumé writers have is an overestimation of what the length of the copy should be. Busy people do not have time to unravel one's family history or marital status and the ages of various children; neither do they want to know the title and date of *all* speeches you've made or articles you've written or workshops you've conducted. The major interests of the one perusing your resumé are your education, work experience, and place in your profession (see Appendix G).

Unless your ego needs it or you are seeking a governmental or competitively top-notch position, your professional resumé should not exceed three pages. (Those persons important enough to be listed in the various reputable Who's Who volumes usually have only about a 20-line paragraph.)

Summary

The serious writer must soon recognize the innate beauty not only of language, but the *proper use* of language. Regardless of the type of communication rendered, it should speak for one's literateness and originality.

Communicating effectively requires study, whether one delivers in writing, speaking, or even evaluating one's own body language. It is imperative to *read, listen,* and *practice.* Unfortunately, both conversation and literature are rife with slang, colloquialisms, trite expressions, "in" phrases (i.e., "let it all hang out," "speaking candidly," "y' know"), and downright sloppy language usage. (I hope, as you've been reading, you've picked up some of mine!).

The prospective clinical professional writer will find it an exciting, enriching experience to look for new ways to express ideas, thoughts, and even scientific findings.

CHAPTER 2: Preparing a Clinical Manuscript for Publication

Getting started on a manuscript is difficult, but you do have one thing going for you—an *idea*. Otherwise, it would not occur to you to put yourself through the exertion of being an author.

Ideas that are good enough to impel you to write about them usually emerge when you think you have discovered something new—a new drug regimen, a new system, a new way of doing something. Or, you may get fired up in favor of (or against) a political or social issue. A chance experience—serendipity—may seem so different and new to you that you want to share it with your professional associates or even the public.

There is the possibility, too, that an editor may have heard about something you have been doing, and will solicit an article from you. You might be asked to present a program or give a speech and, unless you are an old hand at it, you will have to write that out, too. Many organizations request that you submit a copy of the speech beforehand and may want the rights to publish it if they so decide. (If this occurs, make sure that if they decide not to use it, rights will be returned to you.)

If you are in school or taking a course, it is likely you will have to submit a paper or papers during the program.

It is true that the average person does not decide to sit down and write just for his own pleasure.

Getting Started

For most people, the two biggest impediments to getting started are (1) fears about writing ("I've never even written a good letter!"; "I can't possibly write for publication"; "I am no writer — I am a doctor!") and (2) getting yourself to sit down and do it — *and stick with it.* Writing takes discipline and control, and it is very easy to find dozens of other things to do to avoid the task.

11

On the whole, writers and would-be writers have their own methods of production. It is important to decide what period in the 24 hours you are at your peak intellectually and imaginatively. Some people do better early in the morning; others late in the day. And most professionals know their peak times. *Now* is as good a time as any to decide how many pages you can produce in one sitting, and try to stick to that number every day. It is also important to choose the right environment for your highest level of production. The work situation is not usually conducive to writing unless you have a private office or can work in a library. Neither is a busy kitchen or living room where someone else wants to talk or the children want to watch television.

Unless you are an expert with language (and if you are, you are a rarity) you will need resources handy — a good dictionary and thesaurus. If you have already selected the journal you would like to submit the finished manuscript to, have two or three copies on hand so that you can refer to them for things like average length and the "tone" of their published articles. A book on style is useful, too.

Hayes Jacobs, a writer and teacher of note, taught me, "Start writing and keep writing! Write every day and don't let yourself put it off." He also had another suggestion which works for many workshop participants, too. He had the members of his classes submit an autobiography as their first assignment. The reasoning is good. Most people do not find it difficult to write about themselves (a subject they know well) and there is no judgment or grade to worry about. Give it a try. You may find writing easier than you anticipated.

Selecting a Journal

Most professional or health care journals have and try to maintain a specific *focus*. For example, *The American Journal of Public Health* usually contains articles or studies on matters of public health — venereal disease, tuberculosis and other infectious diseases, environmental contamination, rare outbreaks of Rocky Mountain spotted fever, bubonic plague, and the like, and articles on occupational and school health problems. *The Journal of the American Medical Association (JAMA)* concentrates on case studies, research reports in medicine, and organizational news. *Supervisor Nurse* is directed to nursing management problems and some of the solutions to these problems. *Clinical Social Work Journal,* published quarterly, is focused on case studies involving social work with clients or groups. The journals listed here are simply examples. For a more complete list of selected journals, see page 146.

As a prerequisite to making your manuscript outline, one of your best resources is provided by the journals that you feel your article can be submitted to. Scan several past issues for content, length, style, use of photos, tables, or graphs, referencing and such helpful information. Some journals provide details on how to submit a manuscript, others may if you write and ask for instructions; the better book publishers will send you author's guide manuals if they are interested in the material you have submitted (see Chapter 7).

Other Resources

Other valuable resources are reviewing pertinent films, attending workshops or seminars on your subject, and interviewing persons who are involved in similar endeavors or are considered authorities on your subject.

Let's look at an example of pursuing these last three resources. Suppose you are interested in writing an article on contending with the stresses of trying to help hypertensive patients or clients adhere to their often difficult treatment regimens. There are films available either at no or average cost. The American Heart Association, often through its local constituents, sponsors a number of workshops and seminars each year in various parts of the country.

You would interview hypertension research physicians, physicians who specialize in the treatment of hypertension, nurses working in various hypertension clinics, other health care professionals, and patients and their families. One other resource might be to observe in a busy hypertension clinic for a day or two for firsthand impressions.

Before actually beginning work on the manuscript, it is important, perhaps essential, to read the relevant articles published in the previous two years — particularly those that have been published in the journal you wish to submit your manuscript to. This will do more for you than a review of pertinent literature. It will also give you a clue about whether or not the journal published articles on hypertension within that two years. Most journals, except those with a specific focus, are not likely to repeat information they've highlighted that recently.

For all these resources, keep brief but categorized information in your notes.

Preparing an Outline
Now comes the time when you sit down with a pad of paper and your notes in front of you (or maybe you are one of those lucky people who can think on a typewriter) and start to write.

It is very helpful, if not essential, to organize your project in outline form. What is the main focus of your idea? What do you want to get across to the reader? What is the most logical sequence of thoughts you can write down? Maybe you have been doing what some writing instructors recommend and have already started a card file of ideas, pertinent information, references, lecture notes, or written illustrations (anecdotes) on the subject you have chosen.

Maybe you are like some writers and you plan and formulate the general trend of your manuscript while you are driving to and from work, taking a shower, cooking dinner, trying to fall asleep at night.

I know writers who not only do all these things but whenever possible, have a tape recorder along, and when *the* brilliant thought, line, or paragraph comes to mind, they flip on the recorder and tape it.

Whatever planning you have been doing, it should all be there with you when you sit down to really write those first few pages. And your thesaurus, journals, and dictionary should be there, too.

Unless you are a proficient writer, it probably should be a detailed outline. And don't worry about revising it. You probably will, several times, as you progress with the manuscript. Without an outline, your manuscript is likely to come out with a plethora of unrelated paragraphs and will be disorganized. Keep in mind the desired length of the article or chapter and try to stick to that as you do the outline. Sometimes it is helpful to write down your major points and assign them so many lines. And, if you can, make notations where you think subheads would logically fall.

To help you with your outline, make a list of all your ideas, arguments, facts, and illustrations, and then rearrange them in an order that seems reasonable to you and will provide continuity in the manuscript.

The Lead Paragraph

Any editor I have ever worked with has insisted that the "lead paragraph" must "grab the reader and pull him into the story," and I have to agree. I do, however, pull in my horns a little when an author tries to do this by being overly whimsical, dramatic, or "cute."

Let's look at a sample of each:

> Mice are a lot like people. And that includes laboratory mice. For our experiment we had acquired (through someone in the big lab's carelessness), five feisty little males and one equally feisty female. Naturally we each had to name two. I chose Nick and Sadie for mine. Why? Who knows?

And, says the reader to himself, "Who cares?"

Many new writers get carried away with the dramatic approach:

> I will never forget that Saturday night. Six of my patients expired and as I sat in the interns' aerie listening to a dismal, unholy wind rattling every loose pane of glass, I wallowed in my misery and the immense inadequateness I felt. The trees were beautiful, slashing about in the frigid moonlight, but I could only believe they were crackling with disdain at my imagined ineptness.

It is hard for me to suspect that that young doctor really felt badly about his assigned patients dying. If, instead, this character had said, "My God! Is it my fault? Did I do something wrong? Or is it just coincidence?", I think I might feel genuinely concerned for him.

Humor is very valuable when it is well and carefully used. But there is a difference between humor and being "cute." The latter, more often than not, falls flat. The biggest trouble with the "cute" writer is that he overdoes it. I have read a lot of examples of good humor, skillfully interwoven into an otherwise rather serious manuscript. I have read equally as many that leave me cringing.

Nursing students are frequently the victims of an instructor's "wit." The following, from an article in a popular magazine (and I happen to like and respect the publication), is an example of a lead that somehow didn't make me want to read on:

> Some of the most creative and resourceful people I know are nursing students — as they frantically try and come up with the correct answers to tests. (Here the author pats them on the head before taking a whack at them.) It is amazing how much they can teach an instructor who is willing to learn. (Here the author, being nice about the whole thing, rates herself as less than brilliant.) I know I have gotten

information from some of my students in maternity nursing that I couldn't *possibly* get anywhere else. I will bet you didn't know this, for instance — that an orchidectomy is done with a T.U.R. because the orchids are so close to the testicles. I never knew that — and I *gave* the test. But perhaps that is where the term 'deflowering' comes from.

(Frankly, I thought it was an interesting observation on the student's part.)

I am sure numerous people read on, as I did, because there was a great title to the article, and an intriguing illustration. But a little of that kind of humor goes a long way, and the aspiring writer should be wary of attempting side-splitting humor at the beginning.

The lead paragraph should establish the what, where, when, how, why, and who for the reader. If the subject is of interest to him, he will read on. Or, if the lead is clever, he will proceed further before he makes his decision to continue.

More Points on Researching

You have the idea, you obviously know something about the subject, and now you have a working outline. Before you begin to write the actual manuscript, you should find out as much as possible about your subject.

In your search, or review, of the literature, use indexes available whether in or from the major journals in your field. And be sure you look under several headings. For example, if you are a social worker preparing to do an article on counseling unwed teenagers, you would search out titles under "teenagers," "premarital sex," "pregnancy," "unwanted pregnancy," "abortion," and so on. A researcher preparing a study on a certain drug would need to check out the generic name, pharmaceutical information (magazines and texts), and the trade name(s).

And I repeat, when you find the articles or books, read them — or at least skim them thoroughly — particularly if they appear in a journal you want to send the manuscript to. You may find several articles that are very similar to what you have in mind. All too often, an aspiring writer thinks he has the absolute, original idea or method or technique, only to find out it's been covered before — not once, but twice, and even three times. When I was editing for nursing magazines, I was sometimes amused at the query letters we'd get describing some "unique" new method for, let's say, administering a nursing service, and I'd remember that some nurse had instituted the same method years before.

To avoid this kind of disappointment, review the literature and also ask yourself this question: "Even though it isn't a new idea or method or concept, have I developed an innovative approach that *is* different?" If your answer is "Yes", then proceed.

Interviewing Skills

First make sure you know your subject pretty well so that you can ask intelligent and succinct questions. But ask questions relating to those aspects of the subject you're not really clear about.

To interview a busy professional, there are some precepts to keep in mind.

Make appointments ahead of time and explain the reason you wish to talk with them. Don't bounce in unannounced.

If you can, choose the time of day carefully. In a busy hospital, office, or clinic, three periods are bad: first thing in the morning, around mealtime, or late in the day. In fact, these are bad times for any kind of interview, counseling session, or conference.

Also, if possible, pick an appropriate place for the interview — not the cafeteria, not the busy area of work, and not leaning against a wall in some corridor.

These measures may sound simplistic, but they are far from that. They *can* influence whether or not the interview will be worthwhile.

I believe that there are lots of people wiser than I am, and those people can be helpful — and *will* be if properly approached. In fact, frequently the busiest and the most prestigious people are the easiest to approach and are eager to help.

More than once I have regretted not having really listened to wise teachers as I grew up in my profession. Unfortunately, there are a number of others like me.

CHAPTER 3: The Clinical Writing Exercise — Section A

Question Yourself

You're now into serious writing. You've set aside a certain time of day, how many hours you're going to devote to your article or book, your place to write, and you've researched the subject.

Now is the time for a little reflection, a little review, as you sit there with the paper in front of you, and all your notes handy. It is time to ask yourself:

1. Why do I want to write this article or book?
   (Is it publish or perish? Are you really enthused about the idea? Do you want to establish a professional niche for yourself? Is this manuscript essential to a course? A speech?)

2. Do I really believe in what I'm writing about?
   (In other words, do I really want to share some knowledge, a new idea, a solution to an old problem? Have I really made a brand new discovery or, at least, a new, different approach to an old one?)

3. Am I sure of my audience?
   (Do I know who I'm writing to? Do I want to limit myself? Do I want to limit my readership?)

4. Do I want to be simplistic? Grandiose?
   (Do I want the reader to be *with* me as we progress through the story? Do I want to try to prove a scientific point?)

5. Do I want to (and should this manuscript) be formal or informal? A combination of both?

6. What about length?
   (You have three things to consider here: If it is an article intended for a specific journal, review that journal — how long are its articles generally? If you make it too long, be prepared to have a copy editor cut it — and most writers don't like to be cut; it might just be that the copy editor will cut

out the part you like best. If it is a chapter in a book, length should be judged by one idiom: cover the subject of that chapter — don't try to pad it! Don't put too many different subjects in a single chapter — it's better to have short chapters.)

Tables, Graphs, Illustrations

Using tables in an article or book has several drawbacks that make it necessary to review in your own mind whether or not they are really needed — in fact, essential. If not, and if the facts you want to present can be given in the text, it is best to avoid tables.

Readers often resent tables because they are an interruption. Tables take up space and are prone to being dated, in turn, dating your article or book.

Tables should add up correctly, and in round figures, if possible. There are too many astute readers who will soon find out that your figures don't gibe, and they won't hesitate to write you or your editor about it. Headings, tabular material, and comparative facts should be clearly placed.

Number tables or graphs in the order of their appearance. Obviously, Table III shouldn't be mentioned in the text before Table I. Tables should be typed, double-spaced, on separate sheets of paper, and should be placed in the manuscript immediately following the page that you mention them on.

Graphs are, in my opinion, more effective than tables because you can be more original with them — and they attract attention. That is, you can think of illustrative gimmicks for a graph that are not possible with a table. Most of us are familiar with the usual graph illustrations: money is often pictured by piles of coins; population might be lines of human figures, each figure representing so many people; line graphs with shades of grey, black, or other colors are common.

Creativity is possible. If you're writing about how many

apples were grown in the state of Washington between 1975-1980, you can make a line of apples, each apple representing so many thousands of bushels. Or if you want to show how many monitor failures you had in a one-year period on your coronary care unit, monitors in a row are easy to depict. Maybe you have an artist friend who can help you with ideas — and the art.

That brings me to illustrations. When I published my first book, I did the original art work myself. And it "made do" for the first two editions. But I would be the first to admit I'm no artist, and with the third edition, the publisher decided to use a commercial artist to reproduce the same illustrations with more artistic finesse.

There's no reason why you can't develop your own ideas and make sketches portraying them. Your editor can then farm them out for a final rendition. Like written humor, cartoons, used sparingly and well, can add a lot to reader interest. Here is a sample of a slide I use when I lecture on the side effects of the drug regimen a hypertensive has to endure:

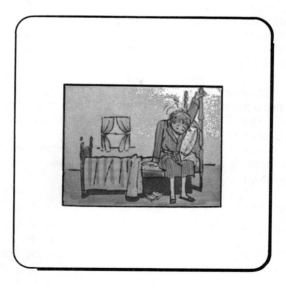

The portrayal here is the first-thing-in-the-morning, hypertensive reaction experienced by many patients with high blood pressure who have to take certain antihypertensive drugs. It takes a long time to get moving.

Halftones

Photographs, or halftones, are very expensive to reproduce — more so if they are in color. If it seems essential to use photographs, they should be originals, although any glossy black and white photo of good quality can be reproduced quite satisfactorily by the printer.

There is no question that illustrations, whether tables, graphs, drawings, or photographs, add to a manuscript. However, the following must be carefully considered: cost, reproduction potential, and — most important — *do the illustrations really add to the article or book?*

Your editor can give you valuable advice and assistance in the selection of art work, and it is wise to discuss art work with him *before* you go to the expense and effort of obtaining your own.

One final thought: don't use paper clips or staples to hold together anything involving art that is to be reproduced. And it goes without saying — **don't** write on the backs of photos or art work. In this day of ball-point pens, all creases and indentations come through when a photograph or other display is reproduced. A felt-tip pen won't mar the front of your picture, but it could smear. The best way is to write on a separate label and then tape or glue it to the back of each illustration.

In a later chapter, we will deal with permissions and copyrights that apply to quotes, photographs, and other illustrations.

Anecdote, Incident, Case Study

The would-be clinical professional writer will undoubtedly be able to provide examples that not only reinforce his point but will help to break up solid text.

In Chapter 2, I recommended that, in making the outline, you should consider the use of anecdotes, incidents, or case studies. Just for clarity, let's define those (with some help from Webster), and give some examples:

anecdote: a narrative, usually brief, of an interesting, often amusing event; actually anecdotes can be used to make a point, as this one does:

> The day after my class on the harmful effects of gossip, one of the class members told me about a conversation he'd heard between two of his class-mates on the bus that morning. Apparently, they had openly discussed the admission to our psychiatric unit of one of the deans of the college and that "he certainly was drunk and obnoxious."

incident: liable to happen; apt to occur; that which happens, or takes place. For example:

> The accident occurred just after mid-night, and the sound of the crash was enough to get me out of bed and to the window. What I saw horrified me. The bus was almost totally demolished, and several bodies were strewn about in the street.

case study: a record of history, environment, and other relevant details (as of an individual) especially for use in analysis or illustration; used frequently by health professionals in both articles and books. Here's the example:

> Mr. B, a 55-year-old businessman, was admitted following his LMD's tentative diagnosis of pheochromocytoma.

25

Rectal temp. 98.8, pulse 102, resp. 22, BP 240/176. Difficulty voiding 30cc dark urine. Foley inserted and Lasix 20 mg. ordered I.V. History of two years moderate to severe hypertension but no marked peaks. Third hospital day BP 240/200. Pt. somewhat disoriented. And so on.

I will not belabor this particular case history, since most, including this one, are long and detailed. But the style should be familiar to physicians, nurses, social workers, and others involved in direct patient care or health education.

In an article (or chapter), all three should be used with care and relative infrequency since, like tables, they tend to interrupt the reader.

Card Files and Tape Recorders

I know of many writers and new authors who firmly believe in keeping an ongoing card file for each manuscript they prepare. One good reason for this is that there are many writing instructors who strongly recommend this method for noting and filing ideas, research data, reference materials, and so on.

My own feeling is that keeping a card file is one labor that can easily supersede the actual business of writing. And that's bad. Under types of writers in Chapter 5, I classify myself as a "procrastinator," and I know that if I had to keep a card file on everything I write about, I could avoid getting down to my article or book for a much longer period of time than I already do.

The exception might be in recording research data, preparing a class paper or research study, when it is important to retain an accurate record of facts or a reference list. Notes, whether written on the spur of the moment, or after you have decided to look up something, can be just as easily woven into the article *as you write it.*

I feel essentially the same way about a tape recorder, although I must admit there have been times when I wished I had one ready to go. A chance conversation with a colleague could set off a whole chain of ideas about the subject you're writing about. Or you may mentally make a rough draft of a chapter or section of an article as you drive back and forth to work, although it's a bit difficult to make notes when you're concentrating on traffic.

Organizing Your Manuscript

In Chapter 2, we discussed preparing an outline. Since review doesn't hurt anyone, I'll again make the seven salient points to consider about your outline.

It should:

1. Contain enough about the main subject to get you started.
2. Establish the what, why, where, when, how and who.
3. List all your ideas, arguments, facts, and illustrations.
4. Sort out these ideas, and put them in order to provide continuity.
5. Place anecdotes, incidents, and humor *where appropriate.*
6. Answer all the questions you and others involved (those interviewed or those who were part of the project) had on the subject.
7. Come to a logical conclusion — make the point you started to make.

More on the Lead Paragraph

It's time to produce several pages. Again, let's review a little on the lead paragraph. It should grab the reader and bring him in. It should be fairly short with reasonably short sentences and it should tell your reader why you want him to read it. Let's look at a sample of a good lead from *Lancet* magazine:

Why *did* Grenadier Thomas Thatcher die suddenly on May 12, 1764, when aged 26 and in his physiological prime? His tombstone by the west door of Winchester Cathedral, raised by his comrades-in-arms as a memorial to his "universal goodwill" and as "a small testimony of their regard and concern," records that drinking cold small beer, when hot, was his undoing: was it the quantity, the quality, or the low temperature which procured such a lethal effect? His comrades summarily rejected the notion that volume alone could dispatch a Hampshire Grenadier; Shakespeare would have been with them, for in *Othello* he declares through Iago that the English "are most potent in potting; your Dane, your German and your swag-bellied Hollander are nothing to your English." No, it was upon inferior quality that the Grenadiers laid the blame, and from which they drew their moral —

"Soldiers be wise from his untimely fall,

And when ye're hot, drink strong or none at all."

I don't know about you, but I was definitely interested in pursuing the story.

Here's an example of a poor lead. The only reason I continued this one was because I kept looking for a period. Virtually the whole lead here *is one sentence* 12 lines long!

As we all have recently had occasion to observe at some tortured length, the elimination of wrongdoing depends on the discovery of wrongdoing, and the discovery of wrongdoing is the business of the press, no less so because critics of the press, who are at least as numerous and clamorous as critics of medicine, have been insisting that the press is not so much the discoverer of wrongdoing as the cause of wrongdoing — a phenomenon that has been around ever since Thucydides reported that messengers who brought news of battles lost during the Peloponnesian War were often executed for their pains.

One further important point about the lead paragraph. It does not have to be written *first.* In fact, some writers block just by thinking about writing an effective lead before getting into a manuscript. If you're comfortable with that, fine — go ahead. As a writer really gets into the article or chapter, he may find himself creating a paragraph that would make a fine lead and may not find it until he's finished the manuscript.

Don't let grammar, spelling, punctuation, or construction get in your way either. For the first draft, just *write!* You'll probably do quite a bit of revising before you're through, anyway. And — even though you *should* know the basic elements of style if you're serious about writing, you can sometimes get an author or editor or English teacher friend to go over it with you editorially. If you can't find such a person, there are professionals who will help you — for a fee.

Once you have a first draft written, or at least five typewritten pages of a first draft, it is sometimes a good idea to put it away for awhile.

Then after some time has elapsed (overnight, a couple of days, a week), take it out and go over it. Does it flow? Can you see where you can eliminate professional jargon? Can you see where you can eliminate the current colloquialisms and insert more interesting, easier flowing language? Here's where the thesaurus can be a big help.

Ask yourself some more questions. Do your ideas follow in a logical sequence? Does the story you wanted to tell make sense as you read it over?

Finally, have someone read it, not for grammar and so on, although don't discourage that person from making notes that will be helpful in such areas. A word of warning: your spouse, lover, or best friend is sometimes not a good choice. They tend to tell you it's wonderful when it may not be; a competitive co-worker will pick it apart. Instead, choose an objective, personally secure professional who is knowledgeable about the subject and you'll get a helpful critique. In fact, an even better way to pick up your own mistakes is to read it out loud to someone. In so doing, you'll find yourself critiquing and formulating better ways to write the material.

Now, if this is only a part of the first draft of an article or chapter, don't try to clean it up to any great extent at this point. Keep on writing. Write five more pages and go through the same process, write until you're finished.

When you have finished and you are relatively satisfied that you have told the story the way you wanted to, then you get to work making it as editorially correct as you can. In Chapters 5 and 6, we will get into the basic elements of style, grammar, and construction, and how to overcome the most common pitfalls in writing.

It is possible, but not probable, that you are one of those rare and lucky individuals who has talent and skill in writing, and you may find you have little to do to the completed manuscript. If that is so, you are fortunate. And — you have become obligated, now, to write more articles and books for publication; in this day and age, we need good and facile clinical professional writers.

A Word About Your Title

You may have already thought of a title that satisfies you but, like the lead paragraph, the title has to interest the reader immediately and impel that reader to start reading.

Long titles are hard to handle. Abstruse titles confuse readers. Clever or cute titles don't often fit in professional journals, although that is beginning to change. Most of us have seen titles involving "games" — games nurses and social workers play with doctors, or games doctors play with subordinates, which of course refer to the manipulating, power playing, and maneuvering that go on in the interrelationships of health professionals (and undoubtedly other professionals, too).

If you are writing a paper that will be read or heard by highly technical, scientific people, your title ought to be seriously clinical and intended for such a select audience.

The title should give the reader a clue to the subject of the article or chapter. In other words, keep some part of the major subject matter in your title (safety, infection control, sex, communications, and so on).

Now let's examine what kind of writer you may be.

CHAPTER 4: The Clinical Writing Exercise — Section B

Types of Writers

There are all types of writers and those of us who labor over — and love — the English language fall into at least a facsimile of some type of writer. I have read about the most famous writers of this century and how they "sit down at the typewriter and work continuously from eight o'clock in the morning until five in the afternoon." I find that hard to believe.

I am a procrastinator and I write when I am in the mood. Admittedly, I have never devoted full time to writing, and maybe that makes a difference. But there have been times when I had the luxury of four to seven days when I solemnly promised myself I would write, and — I end up with an unopened briefcase, a clean house, a clean car, more sleep than I need, and a lot of neglected friendships repaired!

The Procrastinator. It is easy to procrastinate. Too easy. (That's not a sentence, but it makes my point.) Generally, a procrastinator is defined as "a person who puts things off," usually by employing all kinds of excuses. But when you reach your place of solitude, no matter how unpretentious, the wheels begin to spin. The weather forecast says that the next day will be sunny and pleasant but after that, the rain will come. So you say to yourself "Ah, I can mow the lawn, hang the wash outside, and plant the tomatoes while it's nice. Then, when it rains, I will write!" Weather forecasters are sometimes more wrong than right, and it stays sunny and pleasant for the whole four days you have set aside for writing.

Or, you may be an urban dweller. What nicer time to stay in the big city than a long weekend? Let others take to the bumper-to-bumper struggle to the country. You will stay home and write. But — maybe this is a good time to put down some nice, warm carpeting in the bathroom. Or, the third world series game is on and, after all, the series is only once a year. On Sunday there is the newspaper with more words to read than there are in an average length book.

Procrastinators suffer, though. As you begin the frustrating drive back to the real world or as you put down the last section of the newspaper (note I didn't say "very last" because you really can't be more last than last!), guilt begins. You are already past the deadline, and now you can't see any time ahead to get it done. So, you begin formulating excuses.

Procrastinators are not all bad. A surprising number of people work better under pressure and not only do the assigned tasks get done, but they get done well — at the last minute.

The Temperamentalist. I find it a struggle to sit down and write when I am not ready to write. It's a rather weird chemistry that creeps up inside me and I know the time has come. I *want* to write, and once I get myself organized and sit down to write, thoughts begin to materialize into words and, perhaps at 2:00 a.m., I look at the desk, and 10 or 12 pages of manuscript lie there in some sort of a disorganized pile, and I can convince myself I deserve some sleep. If the mood persists, I will likely be up early the next day, and back at my writing with the same enthusiasm.

A "system" like this makes a lot of people nervous — especially teachers of writing who advocate working at least an hour every day — and more, if possible. I rather suspect, though, that some of the best efforts in writing came from a "temperamentalist."

The Bloodletter. There are always one or two students in writing courses who are "bloodletters." They actually *agonize* over a sentence, or the lead paragraph, or even their outlines. Somehow, the instructor will feel that he has failed them — that he made these matters superimportant when they needn't be. The struggle of the bloodletter is real and, unfortunately, it has too often stifled people who might have produced some innovative

34

and interesting articles in the clinical professional field. Many good ideas go down the drain of frustration and that is unfortunate and inexcusable.

To the bloodletter I say: Please! Just write. Write all the things that come into your head, go over your outline, your notes, your observations. There are people out there who can help you — mainly, the editor. The editor who works with your ideas and thoughts will unscramble them for you, will find your lead if you haven't already, and — we hope — will retain your style and originality in the process. If there were not people with good ideas they can't *quite* whip into shape, there wouldn't be any jobs for editors.

The Pedant. Health professionals have been prone to write minutiae with great seriousness and often not only bog themselves down, but take their readers with them. Research writers still do this — and with some justification. But in today's hectic, pressurized work atmosphere, the search is for quick, easy to read, informative, "how to" literature to keep one abreast of one's profession. Although neglect of finer composition is looked on with dismay by students of letters, the clear, succinct, and readable account captivates readers.

The pedant wants to be contemporary but at the same time respects words (bless the pedant!), and this is a perfect niche for the medical writer to place himself in. Review again the excellent lead and style of the *Lancet* editorial quoted on page 28. Intriguing, clever — and contemporary — but well written and with the health professional image intact.

The pedantic writer must be careful, however, that he does not appear ostentatious, didactic, or mired in his minutiae. Some of the more recent books on the Nixon era are guilty of all these faults.

In health matters, careful, informative descriptions of new discoveries and methods, or old experiences made meaningful or renovated, are the speciality of the pedant — the minutiae gatherer. If he can add a touch of humor, he often is the best of all writers.

The Philosopher. People today are looking for some basic meaning to life, and are exploring many realms of human existence. Professionals may be even more sensitive to these things.

The success of science fiction stories has a philosophical basis supporting brotherly love, environmental protection, and a better way of life. Certainly the works of C.S. Lewis, with their strong religious connotations and dreams of a better world, reflect the urgency human beings feel to reach for a nonviolent, support-one-another life concept.*

For the physician, social worker, or other health professional, all the philosophical theories about the process of death and dying have been written, spoken, and argued about at length in recent years. But we should be grateful that it finally has become a part of formal educational programs and is a featured topic on the agendas of most meetings of health professionals.

If you are inclined to write something on a philosophical subject (death and dying, the right to life, abortion, treatment of the mentally ill, organ transplants), you should be able to take a stand on these controversial subjects. You should also be prepared for assault or accolade if it is published.

The philosophical writer, by all intent, should first be a researcher, a scholar. Articles written in the axe-to-grind manner are, of course, partisan, and come off that way to the reader. One of the rules of good writing — whether it is a memo, letter to the editor, editorial, or article — is that a writer should not appear *biased.* That differs from *taking a stand you can defend.*

The Professional Jargonist. Perhaps I have not made a thorough enough study of the literature of academia, which may be why I feel that physicians, nurses, social workers, psychologists, and graduate students in the

---

*Lewis, C.S.: *Out of the Silent Planet,* The Macmillan Co., New York, 1965.

health professions are so guilty of using professional jargon. Of all the poor ingredients that can ruin a good
literary recipe, jargon can most damage an otherwise
potential contribution to health related writing.

Physicians are not as guilty as other health professionals. "Conceptual model" (or "framework"), "crisis intervention," "utilize" (for that good old word "use"),
"behavioral or cognitive objectives," "paradigm," "frame
of reference," "ombudsman," and "logistics" are just a
few of the more traumatizing words you are likely to run
into while reading an otherwise good article or book chapter. Somehow or other, health (and probably other),
professionals in their quest for status feel that they must
"utilize" new and often mysterious words or terms. We
have grown fond, too, of using words that have a ring of
glamor for our speeches and written works; e.g., "clout,"
"accountability," "confrontation," "ping-ponging," and
"impact" or "impacted on!" For a list of jargon, with some
questionable definitions, see Appendix C.

The Laborer.   The would-be author who works hard at
his project is a joy to have in a writing course. This person
does all the assignments — on time — and works very
hard at it. He dutifully sits down at his notes or typewriter
for whatever his self-prescribed time is (an hour or two,
half a day, whatever) and *writes.*

Then he rewrites. Then he uses scissors to either eliminate certain sections or move them around. He is never
happy going to bed with only a few pages done when he's
promised himself he will produce at least eight that day.
More often than not, his final product is disappointing —
slow moving, dull, and with little or no originality. Seldom does he get carried away with elaborate similes like
two I heard from a radio commentator discussing New
York City's financial problems.

First he accused the city government of "dragging its
financial feet"; then he really got daring as he described
the City University of New York as "a giant hulk caught
on the reefs of bankruptcy."

37

When a paper has to be written (class paper, or an article that's been solicited or assigned), it can be listless and without the originality and enthusiasm that make great writers great.

The laborer will emerge with a product that is readable, helpful, and clear. But somehow the reader senses the tiring work the author has put into the article and the reader, too, is tired.

The Gifted Writer. There is ample evidence in the literary world that there is such a phenomenon as the gifted writer — the occasional person who has talent and — "a touch of the muse."

Any talent is a gift, but the reason we admire the talented writer is that he has worked hard to *develop* that talent.

As I have said before — and probably will say again — the good writer has love and respect for language. As Zinsser says in his book, *On Writing Well*:

This is the personal transaction that is at the heart of good nonfiction writing. Out of it come two of the most important qualities that this book will go in search of: humanity and warmth. Good writing has an aliveness that keeps the reader reading from one paragraph to the next, and it's not a question of gimmicks to 'personalize' the author. It's a question of using the English language in a way that will achieve the greatest strength and the least clutter.*

E.B. White, writing on his predecessor as author of *The Elements of Style*, says this:

Will Strunk loved the clear, the brief, the bold . . . . He scorned the vague, the tame, the colorless, the irresolute. He felt it was worse to be irresolute than to be wrong.

---

*Zinsser, William: *On Writing Well. Harper and Row,* New York, 1975, pp. 151.

I believe in color, in imagination, and in revelation (in the sense of revealing something to the reader). And I do sometimes overdo it. It's painful when the editor cuts out those parts in favor of the clear, concise writing that some writing teachers advocate so religiously. I remember once when I was an editor at *RN Magazine* and had kept a diary of a field trip I made to an Indian reservation in Arizona. I was enthralled with that country and wrote the diary that way. Then editor Jack Lavin liked it and used it in an editorial — just as I had written it. I was surprised and pleased.

The gifted writer has ideas and imagination and he *wants* to write about what he feels. He is sensitive to the world he lives in. The health professional who views the physiology, psychology, anatomy, and chemistry of the human body as much more than something he "works with" is likely to want to write about it — and produce a fine and readable manuscript that editors do not have to labor over. Somehow, too, he can spell and use the language in a loving way, and he is careful to check for accuracy when he's not sure.

Most of us have favorite writers, and not all of them write on profound subjects. There aren't many Shakespeares or Thoreaus and perhaps that is good because reading such masters is like making a wonderful discovery.

As potential health care workers prepare themselves for careers, they will find in their readings a physician, nurse, or social worker whose books or articles keep them reading long past bedtime. And they will watch for each new publication that author produces.

CHAPTER 5: The Clinical Writing Exercise — Section C

"Which" Hunts and Other Matters

The elements of style are well covered in a number of texts cited in the Bibliography, but I believe they need reviewing here. There are, for example, a number of pitfalls that even the skilled writer has trouble with, and probably the beginner will stumble into all of them. To repeat an earlier admonition, however, *few rules governing style are infallible*. The exception to the rule occasionally is the only way to go — because it reads better, gets the point across more effectively, and maybe just *feels* better to author and reader. The reader will usually forgive the writer, and more often than not, he won't even know it's not quite correct.

This is not to say the serious writer, beginner or pro, should allow himself to get careless. Using correct form should be a prime concern.

A number of clinical professional journals and most book publishers can furnish their prospective authors with helpful guidelines for style. Certainly these guidelines or manuals save the editor considerable labor and, because of that, save time in relation to when an article or book actually appears in print.

The following list comprises those elements of style, or word usage, that I have found abused most frequently as an editor and a teacher of clinical professional writing. I have not listed them alphabetically, but more in relation to how frequently they occur in unedited manuscripts.

Which and That. The rule I follow with this number one writer's trap is: *which* is almost always preceded by punctuation, frequently a comma. It is a nonrestrictive pronoun.

> Example: The green car that's been following me is gone. The green car, which is very pretty, is parked on Maple Street.

A good test is to read your sentence out loud to your-self. If you hesitate, a comma is implied, and *which* is the better choice. (In fact, this might be a good time for a reminder about most punctuation. As you speak, you automatically — by inflection, voice or tone change — punctuate what you are saying.)

Must and Should. In clinical professional writing these two words are used frequently and interchangeably. Keep in mind that *must* is virtually a command and should be sparingly used.

> Example: A graduate student in social work must interview every member of each client's family.
>> (It is highly unlikely such thoroughness is possible, but the graduate student in social work certainly *should* "interview every member of each client's family," if possible.)

> Example: All personnel assigned to the Code Blue team must respond to the page immediate-ly.

> Example: Fire exits must be accessible at all times.

In these last two examples, *must* is appropriately used.

Finalize. Finalize or any other -ize is part of the current trend to bastard*ize* the language, and it becomes monotonous both to the eye and the ear when it is over-used (and, in my opinion, even once is overuse).

> Example: Finalize the contract as soon as possible.
>> (Make the contract final as soon as possible.)

Omnipotent Words. If you want to get in trouble, use the following:

all	always	every
first	never	none
only	timeless	total

There are some others, but those nine words are frequently abused and should be avoided, if possible. What, for example, is *timeless* except, perhaps, the universe? And even that, you'll note, I've qualified.

Got.   Another abused word, participle of *get.*

> Example: I've got to go *or* I have got to go.
>   (I have to go.)

Upon, within.   Neither of these words should be used unless a specific meaning is intended. *Within* refers to a circumscribed area of space or time.

> Example: Within the Northeast cachement area there are a lot of below poverty level families.
> Example: Upon graduation from medical school, I interned at Cleveland Hospitals.

"Upon" isn't necessary there — *on* is sufficient. It's a good idea, before using *upon,* to ask yourself if you really mean *upon.* Up on what?

Hopefully.   I'd like to just leave it by saying "Hopefully is hopeless," but on rare occasions, it is appropriate.

> Example: Hopefully, they'll get home in time for supper.

I (or we) hope they'll get home in time for supper. (Something or someone has to be hopeful — unless hopefully is used as an adverb, which is its correct usage.)

> Example: We are waiting hopefully for the Giants to win the pennant.

Qualifiers.   Most qualifiers (more, less, a little, very) are not necessary and make for excess baggage.

> Example: I am more tired tonight (More tired than tired — or what?)
>   He is a little taller than Jimmie. (What's a "little'?" An inch? Half an inch?)
>   Vermont is a very beautiful state. (How can it be more beautiful than beautiful?)

Cope. Means to put up with or be able to handle something or someone. It needs *with.*

> Example: If you can cope, you'll make it through graduate school. (Cope with what? Probably many things like the subjects you take, writing a dissertation, inadequate library facilities, and so on — but say what you have to cope *with.*)

Affect, Effect. Often confused by writers and speakers. *Effect* is to make something happen. *Affect* is to have something happen to someone or something. (Exception: psychiatric term for mood.)

> Example: The effect of the change in schedule was an upset student body.
> The students were affected by the change in schedule.

Etc. Means "and other things, or persons" and its use is discouraged by most editors and teachers. Not only does it look awkward and somehow unfinished, but it should be used sparingly, for example, at the end of a list of similar things. The phrase "and so on" or "and others" will suffice.

Farther, Further. These two words are often incorrectly interchanged. *Farther* can be used reliably when referring to distance.

> Example: George's house is farther away than ours.

Further is a time word.

> Example: We can discuss this further (longer, again) in the morning.

All right. The two words are preferred to "alright."

Between, Among. *Among* is used when more than two persons or things are involved.

Example: There was a feeling of dissatisfaction
among the group that didn't seem to exist
between Mary and her brother.

Data. Technically it's a plural word, but use with a
singular verb is acceptable.

Example: The data is being collected by the medical
students.

And/or. A cop-out word combination that is best *not*
used. One or the other usually conveys the writer's
meaning accurately.

Unique. One of the most overused (and incorrectly
used!) words, particularly in clinical writing and speaking.
Defined in any dictionary as "the only one of its kind" —
and how many things can qualify for that distinction?
Unique should only refer to living things — persons,
animals, plants, and the like.

It's, Its. For some reason, inexperienced writers have
a lot of trouble with this, confusing the contraction ("it's"
meaning "it is") and the possessive ("its" meaning
belonging to "it").

Example: It's nice to know its motor will start in cold
weather.
It's (it is) my class day.

CHAPTER 6: The Clinical Writing Exercise — Section D

Tricks and Traps

We've looked at some of the baited traps we can walk into in the ways we use words in our writing. Now let's look at some of the other kinds of pitfalls we can get into if we don't review some rules.

Again, I will leave out some of the less common hazards and concentrate on the errors I often find when critiquing clinical professional manuscripts and books.

Workshop participants sometimes tell me I emphasize words and usage and style too much, and that makes me feel uptight and uncomfortable. But the point I try to make is "go ahead and write it." Pour it all out on paper. Then after it's been on ice a while, weed out the obvious mistakes, the excesses, and the cutesy terms. The reader *hears* what he reads and if he keeps falling over awkward, wrong sounding words and phrases, he'll be tired of, not enthusiastic about, your efforts.

I agree with Zinsser, who writes "...You will never make your mark as a writer unless you develop a respect for words and a curiosity about their shades of meaning that is almost obsessive. The English language is rich in strong and supple words. Take the time to root around and find the ones you want."

I, Me, You, He, Him. Already you see we're headed for danger — when to use certain pronouns.

> Example: John is going to the party with Janie and I.
> (John is going with I?)
> Mary and her will be there.
> (Her will be there?)

Leaving out the other person in the sentence as you read it aloud will help you know which pronoun to use.

Foreign Expressions. Some writers are inclined to sprinkle their stories with foreign expressions, I suspect because it makes them seem like worldly persons. Most of the time, such expressions are incorrectly used, mis-understood, or impatiently skipped over. "Sine qua non" (something absolutely necessary) was a favorite during the Watergate trials. "Raison d'etre" (reason for being) is another very popular foreign substitute for English.

I recall an example of its use in a nursing journal — and a redundant, unintentional explanation of its meaning:

> . . .protecting the public from unsafe nursing care and raising the standards of the profession. These two objectives are manifest today in all we do and serve as the raison d'etre (sic) *for our being.* (Italics mine.)*

Punctuation and Parentheses. Simply put, punctuation is always outside of parentheses unless (1) a complete sentence is enclosed, or (2) an exclamation point or question mark is involved.

Example: No matter how you feel (and I'm still angry), she's going to do what she wants to do.

Example: Margie's youngest (a truly handsome boy!) will be at the dance.

Example: Dr. Brown presented the project to the Academy Fellows who were visiting Philadelphia. (The pathologist, Dr. Williams, was conspicuously absent.)

Single and Double Quotes. When quoting in an article or book chapter, use either reduced type (smaller type, indicated in margin to printer by editor) or quotes at the beginning of each paragraph, but not at the end until the quote is finished. All punctuation is included inside the quote with the exception of a semi-colon. A single quote mark is used when a quote contains another quote.

Example: "As Nixon put it, 'Let it all hang out.'"

---

*Rehder, Katherine E. "1961. . .60 years — A Long Way." *Journal N.Y.S.N.A.*, Vol. 7, No. 1, March, 1976. P. 49.

48

Example: Some of the more frequent complaints were: "A terrible headache"; "A high fever"; "Nausea and vomiting."

Commas. A comma represents a natural, comfortable pause in a sentence. Commas are also used parenthetically — to set off another thought. In a series, some authorities place a comma after each item; some after each item until the last. (I prefer commas after all items in a series, because occasionally, it becomes confusing.)

Example: These are some of the things you'll need, and you won't be sorry you brought them.

Example: That house, old as it is, is a good place for our clinic.

Example: You'll need a thermometer, stethoscope, cuff, and otoscope in each clinic.

Referring to the Subject. The rule outlined by Strunk and White says: "A participial phrase at the beginning of a sentence must (sic) refer to the grammatical subject." Personally, I find this dangling participle lapse charming, and am usually pleased and amused when I find one. This kind of error (and it occurs frequently) is fun to read.

Example: I saw a lot of deer driving down from Vermont the other night.

Example: (from a workshop participant's pretest): A cat is a small animal with four paws, pointed ears, and fur that has nocturnal habits.

Some Miscellaneous Points

Some matters of writing seem miniscule, but are not. They are important. I refer to numbers, abbreviations, and the use of hyphens. Again, there are few specific rules, but there are some helpful guidelines.

Numbers. Although is is best to check style books for proper form for writing numbers, it is generally accepted that numbers from one through nine are written out. From 10 on we use numerals. Large numbers like "a million" can be so described except when writing about sums of money. If a number begins a sentence, it should be written out, for example, "Four thousand people attended the concert, and, according to state police, there were no problems." Or, "Eighteen members of the board of trustees were present."

Abbreviations. In general, abbreviations are not acceptable. As previously mentioned, the abbreviation "etc." should not be used; it is awkward for the reader, whereas "and so on," or "and others" is not offensive. When writing dosages, abbreviations are all right. For example, Morphine 10 mg. or propranolol 80 mg. is understood. Also generally acceptable are Ms., Mr., Dr., and so on.

Acronyms. An acronym consists of the major components of a compound term. The English language abounds with them, and particularly in the areas of health care, and names of government or social departments or organizations. What the conscientious writer has to remember is that the first time he writes about "NIH," he should write out the full title, National Institutes of Health (NIH), immediately following it with the acronym in parentheses. Other examples are American Medical Association (AMA) or American Psychiatric Association (APA).

Once the organization, medical test, government regulation or department has been spelled out — followed by its acronym — the acronym can be used for the rest of the article. If it is a complex term — for example, blood urea nitrogen (BUN), it should be repeated (written out) every couple of typed pages for the uninitiated.

Hyphens. Hyphens are slowly dying out. Most previously hyphenated terms can now become one word, e.g., preoperative, postoperative, nonsupport, or two or three words, e.g., on the job, well written, ill gotten, and so on.

Underlining. Underlining is interpreted by the editor and the printer as italics. Italics should be used sparingly and only for genuine emphasis. (It is usually used for foreign terms, too, and some article or book titles. It is helpful to check the magazines' or book publishers' guidelines for these two uses of underlines.)

CHAPTER 7: The Important Item — Your Style

Writing, rewriting, cutting and pasting, revising, tearing up sheets of manuscript and starting over, reading your manuscript aloud (to yourself, or an objective friend or colleague) — these are some of the agonizing tribulations of the writer. As Hamlet said (and I don't think it was about the process of writing): "(to experience) the thousand natural shocks that flesh is heir to." (Flesh — and mind, too!)

I remember once putting a few pages away and a week or two later being unable to find them. I was frantic because I was sure they were the best, most spontaneous, most impressive pages I'd ever written. (As it turned out, they weren't.)

By now you've developed a *style*. This is the *you* that comes through in your writing. This is the way you express yourself, with ideas, creativity, and language that makes you different from other writers in your field. It may not set you apart to the extent that you'll be recognized "on sight," but the combination of your philosophy, your way of putting words together so that they sound effortless, and your special interest in your subject may prompt people to say about you, "Oh, yes. I've read a lot of the speaker's articles, and they're super."

Maxine Greene, a philosopher who teaches at Teachers College, Columbia University in New York, addressing a dinner meeting with representatives of the American Association of School Administrators, gave her usual fine and compelling message. I've excerpted a passage from that speech because it is so Maxine Greene! I believe I could recognize her exceptional insight and style anywhere.

> When we consider our profession and the young people who are in our charge, we have a responsibility — as never before — to cultivate a critical spirit within ourselves. We have to examine what we

take for granted, to become self-reflective enough to discover whether or not we are structuring our social realities in habitual and conventional ways that may not be defensible at the present time, that may not even cohere with what we consciously believe. Do we, for example, still think in terms of processing children? Do we still blame children for their failures? Do we think of changing children instead of changing structures? Do we listen to children or to parents with points of view at odds with our own? Do we permit others' perspectives, others' ways of talking and seeing, to play into our own? Or do we opt for the exclusivity of professionalism, distributing knowledge in traditional ways, sorting out, distancing, smiling like high priests and priestesses, in the assurance that we know what is needed?*

She sends us a message, as she usually does, and she says it in *her* special way. Her use of language and her deftness with it are illuminating.

One of our problems today (and we have many) is our preoccupation with television, tabloids, the stereotyped styles of popular magazines (including health professional journals), movies, and "second-class" novels. The English language is often ill considered, sloppily used, and even profaned.

What can we do to overcome this preoccupation? First, it is all important to be *observant,* to watch people and things, not just peremptorily, but with concentration to catch the nuances of action and effect. It is also important to be *perceptive,* to understand the meaning of behavior and action and reaction. One does not have to be a psychoanalyst, but by becoming more sensitive, we feel more, and we begin to want to express that feeling. As you

---

*Greene, Maxine. *"Administrators in Troubled Times."* New York, TC TOPICS (Teachers College, Columbia University). Spring/Summer, 1976. With permission from the author.

read this, you are probably thinking, "How can I write a scientific paper that is 'sensitive'?" You probably cannot, but I leave the techniques of that kind of writing to Dr. Notter who handles it with wisdom and precision in Part Two. Review again the "good lead" in Chapter 3. *Lancet* is a well-respected medical journal, and that editorial, after an imaginative beginning, went on to explore the sudden release of catecholamines and its potentially fatal results. Even writers of health profession articles and books can be creative, original, and sensitive, and the contents of those articles and books are read and quoted and remembered.

Travel, whether along city streets or back roads in the country or among other cultures, is enriching. Reading the better works written by authors of the last several decades — F. Scott Fitzgerald, Tennessee Williams, Margaret Mitchell, Carson McCullers, C. S. Lewis, Erma Bombeck, Edna St. Vincent Millay, and Coleen McCullough to mention a few — widens one's creative skills. Obviously, these are some of my favorites, and you may have others. The fact remains, reading will help you write more skillfully.

As you become more comfortable with the task of writing, a style will emerge, sometimes effortlessly.

Rollo May edited the book *Existence,* published in 1958 and still a powerful book. I admire Dr. May's writing, and quote the following to illustrate his compelling style:

> In the ancient Greek and Hebrew languages the verb 'to know' is the same word as that which means 'to have sexual intercourse.' This is illustrated time and again in the King James translation of the Bible — 'Abraham knew his wife and she conceived. . .' and so on. Thus the etymological relation between knowing and loving is exceedingly close. Though we cannot go into this complex topic, we can at least say that knowing another human being, like loving him, involves a kind of union, a dialectical participation with the other . . . One must have at least a readiness to love the other person,

55

broadly speaking, if one is to be able to understand him.*

Thelma Ingles, a nurse whose works I have admired for years, is another skillful and gifted writer. After returning from a long and rich work experience in South America, she wrote an article in *Nursing Outlook,* sharing with us her delight and dismay at the changes she sees in health care — including professional writing:

I am bewildered by the enormous number of new words and the complexity of sentences. What has happened to the simple declarative sentence, clearly expressed? Why do some people believe that quantity is a synonym for profundity and write in elaborate paragraphs what might better be written in straightforward sentences? Mark Twain's rule for grammar — 'avoid surplusage' — is worth remembering.

I am also confounded by the need of some nurses, not to reinvent the wheel, but to paint it another color. The trouble with new or different words to express the old ideas is that the words can give a false sense of progress and disguise history.**

In the second paragraph of that quote, Ms. Ingles goes on to reiterate what I wrote earlier about "unique." What some of today's aspiring nurse authors think is unique is really only the full cycle coming around again. But — one has to be a little older to discern this!

A style that makes its mark may not come easily to most writers. One that does is usually a combination of the gifted, pedantic laborer. If you recall that, in Chapter

---

*May, Rollo, Angel, Ernest, and Ellinberger, Henri F. (Eds.) *Existence, A New Dimension in Psychiatry and Psychology.* New York, Simon and Schuster, 1958. P. 38.

**Ingles, Thelma, "You Can Come Home Again," *Nursing Outlook,* Vol. 24, No. 8. P. 495.

4, I described the gifted as "the occasional person who has talent (and *develops* that talent) and — a touch of the muse.'" Of the pedant, I said, ". . .careful, informative descriptions of new discoveries and methods, or old experiences made meaningful or renovated, are the specialty of the pedant — the minutiae gatherer." And the laborer? ". . .he rewrites. Then he uses scissors to either eliminate certain sections or move them around. . . The laborer will emerge with a product that is readable, helpful, and clear."

An editor is happy (and usually amazed) when he receives a manuscript that shows originality, care, and leaves him little to struggle with.

Students often ask me, "How do you develop style?" There is no easy answer to that, but I would devoutly defend the contention that one must *read,* and read voraciously. Unhappily for our youth (and many adults), television has deprived them of the beautiful world of fantasy, fiction, and truth, the wisdoms of great men and women — the thinkers and the doers who have taken the time to write for us from deep within their special insights.

Magazines, notably the weekly news magazines, have also destroyed the concept of originality. It is distressingly easy to distinguish a paragraph or story that has been lifted from one of these magazines, because, with perhaps the exception of an occasional essay written by an outside contributor, all the columns sound alike to the reader.

Many of the books that are published today and become instant best sellers are carelessly written and leave no lasting impressions. Worst of all, they teach us very little.

"But," you say, "the clinical professional writer isn't writing about things that can be described eloquently and creatively!" I take issue with that.

The writers of this century who became famous and remain so — F. Scott Fitzgerald, Ayn Rand, Mark Twain, C. S. Lewis, Sir William Osler, John Hersey — built history based on history. Today in a forest of literary junk, we are blessed with more good writers like James Michener, Herman Wouk, Saul Bellow, and Carson McCullers.

Honing keen senses of observation and perception is essential to the development of creativity in a writer. Life is forever around us and it is fascinating, curious, delightful — and, indeed, often painful. It is frequently ignored and brushed aside because we are "too busy," the pace is too frenetic for reflection and fantasy. Many people refuse to absorb it, preferring to enjoy the rut they're in — as one writer put it, "A grave with the ends kicked out."

The health care professional who aspires to make a lasting contribution to the literature will develop a style that impresses — once he becomes sensitive to *life*. Who else is as much exposed to tragedy and death and human wretchedness? Who else has as much opportunity to discover and share new knowledge that will help to alleviate these things?

Read, feel, reflect, and take the time to share your life.

CHAPTER 8: The Editorial Process

The manuscript is finished. It is cleanly typed on plain white bond paper with wide margins and, of course, double spaced; you've gone through the "Writer's Checklist" (Appendix B); you've decided on the journal you think it's right for; you've made a copy and filed it (*essential rule number one*).

The Query Letter

A query letter should be written first. Every reputable journal has a "masthead," a list of editors, art directors, production personnel, and so on. Look over that list. If you happen to have met a particular editor, he or she is the person to direct your query letter to. Mention that you've met him and tell him where, i.e., last year's convention, a luncheon, or whatever.

In the query letter, you give the following information (and the letter should not be lengthy):

1. That you have a completed manuscript (and give the tentative title) you'd like to submit for publication.
2. A paragraph describing the article.
3. A paragraph about yourself telling why you're qualified to write it. For example, a physician may write that she's been involved in research on carcinoma of the pancreas for five years, or a psychologist may have worked with developmentally disabled adults, or a nurse may have done a study on preventable accidents in a hospital unit. Also, let the editor know if you have visuals, e.g., photographs, charts, graphs, and the like.
4. A closing paragraph that you look forward to hearing from the editor "in the near future."

It is possible to send several query letters but not advisable. If two or three editors (of different journals, of course) decide they'd like it, what do you tell them? And they're not happy with you when they know you have approached other editors. But — *do not* send a manuscript to more than one journal at the same time (*essential rule number two*).

If, after a reasonable length of time (a month or so), you have not heard anything, you can legitimately write inquiring about the query. Usually query letters are responded to quickly, even if only by a form letter or postcard. The usual procedure when it reaches the editorial office is that the editor it's addressed to shares it with the chief editor, and it may be brought to and discussed at the regular editors' meeting.

If a decision is positive, in other words, they'd like to see the manuscript, the chief editor will assign it to an editor, who will then remain your contact person — your editor. The editor who's assigned to you probably is a specialist in your area.

Mail the original of your manuscript *first class* or even registered mail. Be sure your name and address are on it, and include a brief cover letter. *Copies* of permissions to quote are included, and a reminder if you have illustrations.

Now you *wait.*

Editorial Review

The editor's secretary (or the librarian, or whoever is responsible) sends a card to you indicating the date it's received, its title, and whatever other specific information is necessary. A copy of this card is filed, and your manuscript goes to the assigned editor. Attached to it is an editor's evaluation sheet, with space for comments, and a box to check indicating "Accept, Rewrite, Reject."

In large editorial offices, it is then circulated through the editorial staff. (Some journals have only one editor who makes the decision.) Editors are likely to comment on organization, style, content, value to readers, and extent of interest in the subject matter. Editors do not have time to check the accuracy of dosages, dates, quotes, and references, the spelling of people's names, and so on, so it is *your* responsibility to make sure these are correct.

Once the manuscript is circulated, it arrives back on the chief editor's desk and he or she reads the comments and notes the "score" on accept, rewrite, or reject. If the score is tied, he makes the final decision.

I am definitely on the author's side, even though I spent a number of years as one of those harried editors. I think the author has the right, after a reasonable amount of time (two to four months), to write a letter inquiring about the status of the manuscript. It may nudge the editor.

Rewrite

If the editor asks you to rewrite the article or parts of it, you'll probably be unhappy, because by this time you're bored with it. However, here is one instance where they'll give you a little help. And besides, it's encouraging; it's not outright rejection.

Usually, it indicates (1) they're definitely interested, and (2) there may be a need to clarify some points, or reorganize, or delete, or whatever. Sit on it for a couple of days, and then get to work. It may not be as horrendous as you think. Personally, I'd much rather do the rewrite than have their editors do it. (More on this in the section on "copy editing.")

Here is another time when you may want to enlist the help of a friend who's an editor, a teacher of writing, or an English major.

Rejection

A letter of rejection (or a form letter or postcard), isn't *always* bad news. Sometimes a journal is already planning an issue (to be published three months after they've received your article) on a particular subject, and thus won't be publishing any more on that subject for probably two years. Sometimes they have one or two similar articles already on hand.

And sometimes — well, it just isn't very good.

Unfortunately, busy editors usually don't give you a helpful critique. They simply don't have the time. It is a rare editor who tells you how you went awry. It's up to you to find out your own mistakes. And that's a good exercise.

Don't let a rejection discourage you. Either work the whole thing over (preferred) — or toss it. Neither is easy. But — the editor's points may be well taken — although, in most cases, you won't know what the editor didn't like.

Keep on writing. I'd bet that even the best writers of this century received rejection slips at one time or another. Writing takes stamina, ability, originality, and practice — in that order. And plenty of each!

Acceptance

If accepted, a letter is sent to you, usually right away. That letter may or may not ask a few questions and will request the illustrations. *Always keep copies of illustrations or negatives of photos;* busy art departments can lose materials, too.

Some journals pay on acceptance, others on publication. Some don't pay at all. (Professional journals often don't.) Some offer reprints in lieu of payment.

Unless you are a Hemingway or an author of his note, the publisher retains the copyright. Don't worry about it — it's standard.

And now you wait some more!

One additional note: If an article is timely, i.e., rescue work system in a recent catastrophe such as a tornado or earthquake, it may be published quickly. Otherwise, it could be a year or more before it appears. For example, if you submit an article in August about the treatment or care of poisonous insect or snake bites, it will probably be published in May or June of the following year.

Also, most journals schedule what articles will go in each issue at least six months ahead of time — and sometimes longer. If an issue is already projected dealing with the hospice system in terminal illness, and your article is about working with the families of patients in a hospice setup, yours will be scheduled for that issue.

No editor is going to tell you exactly when your article will be published. It's all but impossible because the mechanics of putting together an issue may make it prohibitive to include yours (space, four-color illustrations, placement, say, in a series, and so forth). Besides, if you tell your colleagues, or Aunt Tillie, or your boss that your article will appear in September and it doesn't — well, it's embarrassing!

The larger professional journals have editorial conferences on a regular basis. Those involved include representatives from editorial, production, art, and the publisher. At these conferences, manuscripts are discussed in terms of which issue they should be scheduled for, what art work will be used (photos, tables, drawings, and the like), whether or not the story should be the lead or cover article, and many other details. Smaller publications have meetings, too, for the same reasons, but with probably only the editor, art and production manager, and maybe the publisher present. Regardless, issues are planned well in advance, whatever the staff or meeting schedule.

Copy Editing. Let's assume your article is slotted for a particular issue. Now it is assigned a copy editor — or, in the case of the small staff, the editor and proofreader. The copy editor goes over your manuscript carefully. What he or she does is usually positive and helpful — reorganization, deleting, sometimes adding, checking some facts, and, perhaps, rewriting. The last item, since I am on the author's side, sometimes worries me, because it can dilute — or even change — the author's *style*. I object to that, and as a writer, I object to it. I want my story to represent *me*, not the copy editor. If, when you receive edited copy, it no longer looks like your "baby," you don't have to accept it. I caution my students not to prostitute themselves for the sake of getting published. I think an author and a copy editor can compromise to the mutual satisfaction of each.

A few copy editors are really frustrated writers. And, in fact, some are good writers. I also believe that my own writing certainly can be improved, and I welcome help. To a certain extent! (Not a sentence, but a point.) Some of the more famous (or infamous, if you will) trade magazines today are being sued by prominent persons for "misquoting" or "quoting out of context." That happens when an ambitious copy editor inserts things he thinks will "sell" or make the article more "sensational."

Nevertheless, many copy editors do a fastidious and excellent job with manuscripts. And even the best, most creative, hardest working writers need their help.

The journal will usually send you an edited copy of your manuscript for your perusal and approval. This is usually your last chance to check your own accuracy — and whether the message you wanted to convey actually comes through.

I urge you strongly not to make drastic changes. This is *not* the time to rewrite. Make only necessary, preferably *brief*, changes. Once the paper is set in type, most journals and book publishers (see the following chapter) will charge you for "author's alterations" beyond a certain specific limit, so only make essential changes — a mistake in dosage, or a proper name, or something that has changed since the editor received the article.

Ask if there's a change in title. Not long ago I heard about a nurse/author who almost lost her job because without her knowledge, the editors had rewritten her title to one that intimidated a physician.

Publication!

I don't need to tell you much about publication. To put it blandly, it's nice. It feels good when the issue arrives — maybe an advance copy — and there's your name *in print*. It may have happened before, and it may happen again, but it feels good.

Your friends and colleagues will congratulate you. Your bosses will look favorably on you. You'll get invitations to speak. Other publishers may approach you.

Enjoy it all. It's hard work, this writing business. And — it is uniquely you.

CHAPTER 9: Some Points About Book Publishing

Basically, writing a book involves all the rules of grammar, outlining, gathering the facts, correct referencing, and so forth. Getting a book published involves some differences, and in this chapter, we'll cover those differences.

The first, considerable difference is the time it takes. It takes a long time to write a book; it takes dedication, and the ability, if you will, to forego *fun* for awhile. It takes postponing other matters that should be taken care of.

People normally write books because they want to, not because they have to. And they want to for a variety of reasons. Perhaps a potential book author wants the material of his thesis or dissertation to spread further than on microfilm in some university library. Or a lengthy research project has produced results that should be known outside research circles — notable example, the Kinsey report.

Whatever the impetus, it's there, and a query letter is in order. There are several reputable book companies in this country that specialize in texts for health professionals and some are listed in Appendix F.

The query letter is essentially the same; i.e., it contains information about the subject(s) covered, the author's background, the proposed length, the potential market or audience, and what you can send for the editor's review.

What you should send are: (1) Tentative chapter headings with a brief abstract of what each chapter will contain; (2) a foreword or introduction outlining the purpose of the book, and the potential market it is directed to; and (3) at least two sample chapters. The last item doesn't necessarily mean Chapters 1 and 2. Any chapter will do. The purpose of sending several chapters is threefold. First, it gives the editor an idea of the validity of your writing. Second, it gives him an idea of your style. And third, it tells the editor whether or not you can write. If a chapter is badly organized and grammatically incorrect, it means too much and too costly an effort for the editorial staff.

Your manuscript should be as clean as possible, properly referenced, and you should *keep copies*.

The material will be reviewed by the editors, and many publishers send it (without author's identification) to reviewers who know the subject. When all these evaluations are in, the editors make a decision to accept, reject, or ask for a revision or rewrite.

Briefly, a rejection or rewrite doesn't necessarily mean it's all bad. There's the concern of the publisher that the potential market isn't worth it. In these days of tight economy — which is likely to continue for a long time — publishers are wary of putting out a book that may have a very limited audience.

The Contract
Thinking positively, let's say it's accepted. Sometimes the book editor will meet personally with you. Sometimes the details are worked out in the mail. The details involve a contract. Most book publishing contracts are essentially the same — a lot of small print with a lot of detail that's unlikely to apply to health professional texts; i.e., texts on family casework or surgical procedures — hardly a case for movie or television rights. However, if it's your first such contract, it's wise to let a lawyer look it over.

What you do need to note includes the following items. First, the working title. It is understood by both parties that it may change. Second, the projected date for finishing the book — in other words, the deadline. A deadline is important because it nudges your conscience to finish it on or before the due date. Fortunately for procrastinators like me, this deadline is not engraved in stone, and publishers can be somewhat flexible — to a limit.

Third is terms for payment. Unless you are an established author, the current rate is usually between 10 and 15 percent per copy royalties for the author. Few health professionals make any significant amount of money from a textbook, unless it's a book with a general public as well as a health professional audience (example, William Nolan's *The Making of a Surgeon*).

Consider carefully the timing of your book's publication. It is worthwhile to publish early in the year because the date of publication makes your book new or recent. For people compiling bibliographies or looking for references, that's important. You and the publisher should try to get the book out close to the dates of your discipline's major professional convention(s) so that it gets prominent display in the exhibit area.

Royalty Payments

Usually, royalty checks are issued twice a year for the first two years after publication. If your book survives beyond that (and some do for many years), you will receive your royalties once a year. (These checks are declarable income tax items.)

Revised editions should be mentioned here. If your book is "paying for itself" or better, you'll probably be asked to produce a revised edition about every four years. These revisions are sometimes minor, sometimes major, depending on the subject, the progress in your professional field, and so on.

Permissions, Copyright, and Other Particulars

It is a revelatory experience to read the words of the creative writer. He ascribes "fury" to a tornado, "stillness" to Appomattox, "thought" to a bird. Witness the master, Will Strunk (on style): "Writing is, for most, laborious and slow. The mind travels faster than the pen; consequently, writing becomes a question of learning to make occasional wing shots, bringing down the bird of thought as it flashes by." (*The Elements of Style*, p. 62.)

The manuscript is yours, but if you've borrowed from others who are masters (as I have a number of times in this book), you must give them credit. Since most publishers who accept a manuscript also assume the copyright, you have to write to the publisher of the material you've "borrowed" for permission to quote from the book or article. This is a good idea even if you paraphrase the quoted material. Remember to include in your letter the quoted material exactly as it will appear in your article or book. It is not essential to get the author's permission also, but personally, I prefer to do that as a courtesy (see footnote of Appendix A).

The general rule is that you can quote up to 200 words of another author's article, speech, or book without permission, but my advice is that you should request permission anyway. A sentence, or even a few sentences, can be quoted as long as you ascribe them to their creator; e.g., "according to Strunk and White in *The Elements of Style* ... "

Even though you are not likely to be involved in obtaining copyrights, it's a good idea to know the process. It is relatively simple. If you have questions about copyrighting, write to: Register of Copyrights, Copyright Office, Library of Congress, Washington, D.C. 20559. If you want to copyright an article, book, course outline, or whatever, request the appropriate form, fill it in (including the title, author(s), name of the publisher, and date), and enclose the required fee.

A written work is said to be "in the public domain" (i.e., not necessary to reference or get permission), if it comes from a government publication, the copyright has expired, or it has never been copyrighted. (As to the last, I'd still advise getting permission if the author is living.)

If you use a direct quote (exceeding 200 words) in something you're writing for publication, you need to obtain the publisher's permission. Most publishers are happy to give permission — as are most authors — but will send you a credit line to follow conforming to their style or requirements. The line should be used in its entirety.

Beware of using too many references. Many times, in editorial offices, I have heard this comment — or seen it written on an editor's evaluation form: "Twenty-two direct references? What, in these 16 pages, could be original with this author?" We know, and you will read more about this in Part Two, that technical and class papers, masters theses, doctoral dissertations and the like must contain considerable reference material, including a "survey of the literature."

For a magazine article, unless it is highly technical, a few choice or necessary references are okay; the reader still recognizes that he is reading *your* work, as shown by your original writing style.

Be Careful What You Write

Because there is some connection to the previous section on copyright, we should briefly look at plagiarism, slander and libel.

Plagiarism. Strictly defined, plagiarism means to pass off as your own the ideas of another. You can get into serious trouble — and so can your publisher. Some authors do this intentionally, thinly disguising another writer's already published work, or part of it. It's not easy for the editor to spot, but the original author certainly will. Some would-be writers actually "lift" entire sections of published material and offer it as their own. Legal trouble can be the result.

Slander. Slander is defined as speaking about someone — or something in a defamatory way. If slander can be proven (by witnesses), you can be sued. Some years ago, I sat in an audience of well over a thousand professional people, and listened to a physician publicly criticize a mental institution he had visited the week before. Besides airing his views to the audience, his talk was being recorded. The administrator of the named institution quickly received word of the derogatory comments, and the physician barely missed being taken to court.

Libel. The dictionary defines libel as: "The action or *crime* (italics mine) of injuring a person's reputation by something printed or written or by a visible representation." Frequently we read about lawsuits brought against

71

sensational newspapers, or porno magazines and films, and in several instances, persons have been awarded substantial damages for libel.

A word of caution: Be careful what you write about a living person, especially if it's to be published. If what you write casts aspersions on a person's character or insinuates anything damaging about him, it makes you liable to libel. However, even if such an intimation does appear in your manuscript, the publisher or editor will probably catch it. He is partly responsible for what appears in print in his publication, and does not knowingly take that kind of risk — nor should you.

Class Papers and Speeches

Would-be authors in all the health care disciplines seem to have the feeling that a class paper that rated an A-plus (particularly when the instructor has penciled a note at the end, "You should try to publish this") should be published *as is.*

Here is an instance where the query letter should indicate it is a class paper, and that you will revise it before you submit it. Class papers are seldom read with enthusiasm by the average busy editor.

Revision of a speech, on the other hand, requires a minimum of effort. Obviously, you must eliminate such introductory remarks as how happy (or honored or privileged) you are to be the speaker. Your "warm-up" joke must go. Reference by name to the group you're addressing may be of no interest to the reader. And your closing remarks can, for the most part, be eliminated with no loss.

If your manuscript has been adapted from a speech you've given, however, you should keep two important points in mind. First, make sure that in your correspondence with the sponsoring group, they have not indicated previously that they want publication rights to your material. Second, be sure you give, in a properly annotated footnote, the source of the article, namely: title of your talk, sponsoring group's name, date and place of your presentation. Precede all that, of course, with, "This article is adapted from a speech . . . ."

References and Bibliography

Books, in particular, need references and a bibliography. (Most novels don't unless they are historical.) For more technical articles or those citing others' research, references and a bibliography may add a lot to the validity of your manuscript.

To clarify (and there are new writers who don't know this), references *refer* to specific passages that should be reproduced exactly as they appear in the original version — duly credited.

The bibliography is a list of books and articles the author has read and studied that have shed more light on the subject for him and will do the same for the reader. He has broadened his knowledge by reading what other authors have had to say about the subject.

How to set up your references and bibliography (including how they're numbered) differs from one journal to another, and is also true among various book publishers. Your best bet is to look up reference lists in the journal you are submitting your article to, and review their specific style for such lists. For example, a social worker who has prepared an article for *Social Casework* with several references and also wants to add a short bibliography, consults that journal and follows its style.

Several book publishing houses I'm familiar with have authors' guides that include much helpful information — including their preferences for documenting background material. Among these publishing companies are Harper and Row, Prentice-Hall, and Van Nostrand Reinhold. Your book editor-to-be will be happy to send you one without cost.

Check for Accuracy

In line with the preceding section, let me repeat my earlier words of caution regarding accuracy: make sure you check *all* your facts and figures, particularly medical terms, dosages, spelling, generic names of drugs if any, and, in the case of references, the exact page number(s) you're quoting from.

It is the rare editor who has the time to research all such materials, even though he or she is responsible for accuracy as much as the author is.

Appendixes are very desirable in nonfiction books, particularly a how-to textbook. Note what I have included in this book (with sources duly credited where necessary): a list of journals in the major health care fields; a sample of editorial marks; a sample resume; a list of transitional phrases; and other matters pertinent to writing.

Whether or not to use a graph, table, list, or other aid within the text of your book or to add them as appendixes depends on how important it is to have the visual aid close to what's being written about it. And the publisher, because of editorial or production preference, may not agree with where you want the visual aid placed in the body of the text. (In that case, I'd go along with his decision.)

Indexing

Indexing is not nearly as difficult as it is reputed to be. There is always the exception, of course, and the exception here is the long, complex text (e.g., the enduring Cecil & Loeb volumes on medicine). I have used (and paid) librarians to do some of mine; there are also free-lance indexers who are very thorough — for a fee. Sometimes the publishing company will arrange to have a professional indexer do it for you.

I have found a relatively simple method of indexing in preparing my books, and do it myself with a friend's help. It usually takes only a few hours for an average-length text (350 to 450 pages). Several publishers, in their author's guides, suggest indexing on three-by-five cards as you go along, putting down the main headings and adding page numbers after you receive the final page proofs.

I find it easier to have a friend (yes, you *can* do it alone, but it takes longer) write down on a large pad all the letters of the alphabet (capitalized), leaving sufficient space. Then I go through each numbered page proof and wherever I see an item referred to directly or indirectly I tell the friend and give the page number.

Once you've done that, you alphabetize all the subentries. Type your index double-spaced — usually 25 entries to a page, depending on the physical size of the book, number the index pages and it's done.

> Example: Case histories, preparing
>   clients' participation 76-78
>   social worker interviews 79-86
>   physician input 87-90
> Nurse practitioner, role of
>   in independent practice 152-154
>   in rural setting 126-136
>   in urban (inner city) setting 137-151

Author's Biography

Whether your effort is an article or a book or a speech, the editor needs to know something about you and your readers want to know, too.

I feel the same way about an author's "blurb" (usually listed under the heading, "About the Author"), as I do about a professional's resume: it needn't contain every detail of your life. Imagine this one in a medical text: She (the author) is married and has three children. She knits and crochets in her spare time, loves tennis and skiing, and is an excellent cook.

I can't quite see what this has to do with her expertise for writing the book! I would like to know her educational background, her experience, and what aspects of her work accord her to be an authority on the subject. Previously published works can be mentioned, as well as any *outstanding* honors.

It is in this blurb, too, that acknowledgments can be noted of those colleagues who had a significant part in a project, or offered considerable help with the manuscript.

CHAPTER 10: What It's All About

This is a small book. Most books about writing are small. (Strunk and White is only 78 pages and fits in your pocket.) One of the exceptions is the excellent volume, *The Careful Writer*, by Theodore Bernstein, a fine book and well worth inclusion in any writer's library.* (Incidentally, the use of "that" and "which" is handled in detail in Bernstein's book, pp. 443 to 446.)

We intended our book to be small, but we also intended it as a kind of quick reference for the active, industrious health care professional. Between us, we've had 25 years of editorial experience on various journals, and both of us have published books and numerous articles. This is only to tell you that we know the pitfalls; we know where health professional writers can get into trouble.

There are few professionals who make a lot of money for the written works they labor over. But they can and do make worthwhile and useful literary contributions to health care and to their colleagues in their own and other disciplines. The ultimate attainment, happily, is that the sick, the hurt, the destitute, the disturbed, the old, and the young will, in the last analysis, be the beneficiaries.

In my head, and I'm sure in Dr. Notter's head, too, that's what it's all about.

Speaking the English Language

To those of us who have made an effort to write seriously over the years (and I suppose I have to add, those of us who are older!), the spoken language today is appalling. I hasten to add, however, that we are as guilty as the next. My father used to tell me frequently, "Two wrongs don't make a right," and I admit I still agree with that axiom. Because we *speak* weird English every day doesn't mean

---

Bernstein, Theodore: *The Careful Writer*. Atheneum, New York, Rev. Ed., 1975.

we have to write it, especially in a clinical professional manuscript. Sure, it's appropriate in a trade book or magazine. And I would advocate that the beginning clinical professional writer, in particular, write it down as it comes into his or her head. There is time later to rewrite the manuscript in a clear, concise, and *correct* style.

Try this simple exercise. Rewrite the following sentences that represent English(?) as it is commonly spoken today:

> Don is into tennis in a big way!
> Let's update the project and finalize it.
> I don't know where it's at at this point in time!
> The new president is determined to do his own thing.
> Lay it on the line, Doc. Is the patient gonna make it?
> Where are you coming from?
> Hopefully, the name of the game is money.

In the process of changing these into *simple* (and lasting) English, make note of the punctuation, too.

As I've said many times, the rules of grammar and writing are not engraved in stone. There are a number of gray areas — figures of speech that are acceptable today would have caused a journalism student of yesterday to fail the course. We've reached a happy medium — e.g., using the first person rather than the stilted, "The author thinks . . .," or "My colleagues and I believe . . .," and ending a sentence with a preposition instead of wending your way through "with whom or with which I worked." It sounds smoother to say "I worked with."

What is important and what distinguishes you as having an individual style comprise the sounds you make on paper. You reveal yourself as an *individual*; you make your mark because you are you.

What do your written words tell people about you as a person? Do you sound autocratic? Stuffy? Unexciting? Unsure? Or, do you sound comfortable? Humanistic? Like a sage or mentor? Like someone the reader would like to know, study with, seek help from?

It is dangerous to "overwrite" or adopt contemporary colloquialisms to make an impression. Neither serves to promote clarity. I tried to make that point on page 16 in the intern's description of his feelings after six patients under his care had died.

When you have formed the habit of reading the works of the better writers of today and yesterday, there is a temptation to mimic or copy their styles. But, eventually, you'll fit into your own mold, and the prior experience of imitating can only be enriching.

An Exercise in Self-Exercise

I'm not at all sure there is such a term as "self-exercise," but I like it and it fits what I'm about to advise.

Let's say that, after reading this far, you're still convinced you can't write, haven't the time to write, will never be published, or haven't anything of interest to say. (If any of those is true, I've spent untold weeks in a futile effort to convince you otherwise!) I would not go on record as believing *anybody* can write, any more than I'd make the same claim about being an engineer, pathologist, painter, or anything else.

But I *am* convinced that there are those in the health care professions who have the background, the ingenuity, and the talent to contribute to the future of medicine, nursing, psychology, social work, and so on, through the written word. If you'll recall from the introduction, I teach clinical professional writing. I haven't taught a single course wherein at least a few of the students haven't had real ability, a feel for words, organization, and clarity. More than a few go through the self-exercise of working on a paper only to put it aside for all the reasons we know so well. Some, to our mutual satisfaction, have been published. It is disheartening to me that a number of promising manuscripts now lie filed away somewhere. But I'm optimistic — someday they'll be worked on again.

Let's look briefly at a self-exercise that you can do privately and at your own pace. Select a subject — any subject — that is of more than mild interest to you, and sit down (when you have some time to spare), and write about it. Try to follow the rules, number one being JUST WRITE. Tell someone out there how to do it — how *you* did it. Or, select a clinical professional subject that you want to know more about, e.g., the correct measurement of central venous pressure (CVP) in the recovery room. Go out and interview the anesthesiologist or certified registered nurse anesthetist or emergency room physician.

Take careful notes and write a how-to article that will help all the people involved in CVP in the recovery room, intensive care unit, or wherever CVP is necessary. Just write it as a self-exercise in pulling interview material together. Most clinical professionals don't mind being asked questions (as long as you adhere to the rules — right time, right place, and, preferably by appointment).

Another self-exercise: Read an article or a book and then sit down and write a rough review of it. Make outline notes as you read — they help, and also provide a method for schooling yourself to pick out the important messages that the article or book reveals. This kind of manuscript may never be seen by anyone but you; nevertheless, the more you practice this self-exercise, the more comfortable you'll become with writing and with yourself.

EPILOGUE

In Part One, I have tried to give the aspiring clinical professional writers important, basic details that are necessary to get himself or herself published. I've told them how to proceed. Dr. Notter and I have given them bibliographies for obtaining further information. Now it's up to the writer.

Dr. Lucille Notter is referred to by many — at least in nursing — as "the dean of research writing." I admit I know little about it and that's why I asked her to help me with this book. Part Two, on research writing, follows. It will help anyone involved in writing a research report or submitting a grant proposal.

PART TWO

It is with sincere appreciation that I acknowledge the contributions of Marguerite C. Robey, R.N., Ed.D., Chairman, School of Nursing, Union University, Jackson, Tennessee, who read the manuscript of Part Two, and whose comments were most helpful.

Lucille E. Notter

CHAPTER 11: Publication of the Research Report

It has frequently been said that a piece of research has not been completed until it has been reported in the literature. Perhaps the statement bears repeating here to emphasize the need for better communications among scientists in the health professions. The need is also especially apparent between the scientists who are doing the research and the clinical practitioners who should apply the findings. It has been said that the scientist or researcher writes for and communicates mainly with other scientists or researchers interested in the same highly specialized problems. Although it is true that there is a place for the detailed research report aimed at the research audience in a particular field, researchers also need to be able to write simpler reports for the broader audience in their own clinical field and across related disciplines. The chapters in this section will deal with the writing of research reports for both audiences.

There is real value in preparing more popular types of articles for either professional journals reaching members of the health professions who are not skilled in research methods, or popular nonprofessional journals having a very general audience. Articles for the latter may be written in addition to those prepared for the scientific journal. They are usually presented in much more simplified form depending upon the sophistication of the journal's audience. Since Part One of this book has been devoted to writing in general rather than the writing of articles reporting research, Part Two is devoted to a discussion of the scientific report rather than the "general audience" article.

Although not all research is well done or relevant to the work of health professionals, that which is well done and important should be available to the audiences needing the information. Progress in health care depends upon all health professionals — physicians, nurses, social workers, nutritionists, health educators, and others — having access to the new knowledge generated by research that is of value to them in their work.

Health care professionals doing research, particularly large-scale research, may find that their work generates publishable data at various stages of their investigation. Longitudinal studies, such as the National League for Nursing's Nurse Career-Pattern Study, in which data are collected on nurses at 1-, 5-, 10-, and 15-year intervals following graduation from nursing school, can be the source of a number of articles and monographs.* Multi-faceted studies, such as the investigation of health care behavior and experience of residents of East Baltimore under the auspices of the Health Services Research and Development Center, Johns Hopkins Medical Institutions, also provide data for more than one report. The latter study is part of a larger investigation of health care groups who use three different care systems. It involves three sample populations: enrollees in an HMO, the general community, and public housing project residents.** However, most commonly, the investigation produces data that can be adequately reported in a single article and should reach those who need the data while it is still current. A report of research completed five or six years before it is submitted to a journal will not be as welcome to the editor as it might have been at the time the research was completed.

Keep in mind that the size of the investigation and the number of papers it generates are not necessarily the most

---

*See Knopf L.: Graduation and Withdrawal from R.N. Programs: A Report of the Nurse Career-Pattern Study, DHEW Publication No. (HRA) 76-17, Washington, DC, Government Printing Office, 1975. Lucille Knopf: Debunking a myth, Am J Nurs 74:1416-1421, Aug. 1974.
**See German PS, Skinner EA, Shapiro S: Ambulatory care for chronic conditions in an inner-city population, Am J Public Health 66:660, July 1976.

important aspects to publication. An article which reports on a relatively small but well planned study may serve to stimulate additional research in a given field. Scientific progress can result from an aggregate of small studies as well as from larger, more sophisticated types of research.

If as noted above, a major factor in publishing research reports is the desire to contribute to improvement in health care by communication of relevant findings, then the need for this communication is the most important reason for writing and publishing the research report. However, it is recognized that there are other factors that may influence the desire to publish. For one, the study may be financed by an agency under an arrangement that includes publication, or the researcher may be a member of a faculty requiring publication — the publish or perish phenomenon.

Decisions about Publication

As a prospective author you have several modes of publication to consider. Publication of a book, also sometimes referred to as a monograph, may be your first choice because you wish to present the research in considerable detail. The terms books and monographs are often used interchangeably. A book is usually called a monograph when it presents a treatise or a highly detailed and documented study in a limited subject area. Monographs considered to be of value in the scientific community are often published by university presses, professional associations, and foundations. However, preparing a book for publication takes time, sometimes more time than you as the researcher want to use before communicating your findings. Therefore, you may decide, especially if the research is timely, that the scientific article is the preferred way to reach your audience while the material is still current. Of course, you may decide to do both: write one or more articles and also prepare a book or monograph for those who will want much more detail about the methodology and data analysis.

The Book or Monograph

Publication of a book or monograph is a major undertaking. As noted previously, the scientific monograph type of report is appropriate when the audience is made up of scientists interested in the details of the research, that is, a complete report of the work done. Graduate students, especially those working on doctoral research in the same or similar areas, also will be an interested audience. Much important work is reported as monographs for these groups and they make a valuable contribution to the literature of science and to progress in the scientific effort.

Monographs include a discussion of the problem studied, a broad discussion of the literature pertinent to the study and which provides the rationale for it, and a discussion of the hypothesis or hypotheses that guided the study. A chapter may be devoted to the theories basic to the study — the conceptual framework. The research method will be described in another chapter in sufficient detail so that the work can be adequately evaluated or replicated by other scientists. The method of data collection, the data obtained, and its analysis may be spread over several chapters, depending upon the complexity of the methods used. Final chapters will be devoted to conclusions drawn and implications of the research for further study or for clinical practice. Appendixes usually include additional data not presented in the text (for example, raw data may be placed here when this is indicated) and tools used in carrying out the study (checklists, rating scales, questionnaires, tests, and so forth).

In many instances monographs are of great importance to the scientific community. They are costly to publish, they are not necessarily best sellers, and they do not always produce royalties for the author; however, they are needed. Scientists in the health field are alert to this need and work persistently to promote the interest of associations, foundations, and others, including commerical book publishers, in the publication of important research as monographs. Commercial publishers do occasionally produce book-length research reports that appeal to a limited audience as a public service, but it is understandable that more often they are interested in serving a broader audience with general professional interests.

The goal of reporting research in a book written expressly for the broader audience is not necessarily inappropriate. If the report is written to interest and be read by a larger audience, it may have greater imapct on practice. In this case the language of the report may be simplified somewhat and the focus may be more on the findings and their implementation, although sufficient detail regarding the methodology and data analysis may be included to indicate the quality of the study.

The Article

One of the most important, valuable contributions to the advancement of progress in health care has always been the journal article. In contrast to monographs or books, articles are brief and hence more quickly written. They are thus able to bring important research to the attention of the profession while the findings are still current. Then, too, articles usually reach a larger audience, depending, of course, on the circulation of the journal. Finally, articles can be more quickly read by the interested but usually busy person. In this section the major emphasis will be on some of the steps involved in the selection of a journal. Later chapters will deal with planning and writing the research article.

Essentially the same procedure is followed in selecting a journal for the research report as for any other type of article; the preferred audience and the nature of the content are the major determinants. For this purpose, familiarity with the scientific journals in the field will be an asset. If you are not familiar with them, browse among the journals in a medical or health science library or talk with professionals who are familiar with them. If the article has been solicited by an editor, the problem is slightly different in that, in this instance, you must decide if the particular journal will provide the best outlet for the audience you wish to reach. If it does, then you are in a stronger position than the author who has to select a journal and approach the editor.

Authors in the health field have a variety of professional journals available to them. Although some of them, such as the *Journal of the American Medical Association* and the *American Journal of Nursing,* publish general content, many others are specialty journals, limited in the scope of content in which they are interested.* Your choice of a journal will be determined by the area of research it features. If your research is in some aspect of coronary care, you may choose a journal devoted to this specialty or one devoted to general content in a particular health care discipline — nursing, medicine, dentistry, pharmacy, nutrition, and so forth.

Having selected a journal, you may elect to write to the editor describing the proposed article and its purpose; or, you may decide to take a chance and submit the article without having first determined interest in it. The latter is more risky and therefore not the preferred method. However, it is often the method used, particularly if the paper has already been written for some other purpose and is ready for consideration as an article.

Decisions about preparing an article for a particular journal often are made by talking with editors at professional meetings, such as the annual convention of a professional society or organization. The would-be, less well-known authors in the health sciences field can use these opportunities to meet editors and learn about their current special interests, as well as to become better known themselves. When editors express interest in a proposed research report, they can be most helpful in giving the prospective author ideas about how to focus and develop the article.

---

*See Bibliography — Part One for a list of journals in the health fields.

Whatever is done to select the best journal to publish the report of your research, it is unethical to submit your manuscript to more than one editor at a time. The correct practice is admittedly slower but, if the article is well written and on a topic of interest, and if sufficient care has been taken to select the right journal and to determine interest in advance with the editor, there will be reasonable assurance that the manuscript will be accepted. If it is not accepted, then, and only then, should you submit it to another journal.

CHAPTER 12: Planning the Scholarly Research Article

Anyone starting out to write an article needs to have a general plan before sitting down to write. Not only does the author need to consider the journal for which he is writing, but he needs to decide on the content and on the way he wants to present it. For researchers, the decision of how to present the content would appear to be relatively easy: the nature of the content is largely determined by the research already done.

Most publishers have a style sheet or manual which can be helpful in suggesting the general format of articles in their periodicals. These guidelines for prospective authors may be published periodically in the journal or may be available upon request. In planning an article, it is wise to become thoroughly familiar with the guidelines and general format of articles in the journal selected. Although research reports or scientific articles usually follow a particular format, there is also considerable variety in their presentation. Editorial and personal style enter into this variety and these will be discussed in the next chapter.

The selection of the content itself within the general framework of the journal's style will depend upon the focus the writer selects. He may elect to present a straight-forward report of the study beginning with its purpose and ending with a discussion of the findings. On the other hand, his focus may be on some other aspect of his investigation, for example, the methodology used, the theoretical or conceptual framework guiding this and similar research efforts, the findings, or a review of the literature of research in the general area of interest.

Articles generally are relatively short in length and therefore cannot cover all that was read, all of the decisions that had to be made, or a detailed account of a fairly complex research method. Sometimes only one facet of the research can be covered adequately and others must be left for later articles. Once the decision has been made as to the content to be presented, the next step will be organization of the material.

Organizing the Content

A major problem of inexperienced writers is organizing the content. Poorly organized material, whether its cause be lack of an outline or fuzzy thinking, can result in hard sledding for the reader and ultimately in very poor communication. Well organized material following an orderly progression of thought will lead the reader through the research with less effort, more interest, and better understanding. Logical organization of content, together with a readable style, are essential to the goal of all scientific writing: to accurately inform others about something the author considers important.

Although some experienced writers develop articles without a written outline, many do jot down at least a brief list of the major areas to be covered. Many also note the ideas they want to include within these major areas and they continue to add to these ideas as they think of them prior to actually writing the article.

An outline for a straightforward research report will often include the following elements: an introduction, a review of the literature, a description of the research method used and of the study sample, an analysis of the data obtained, and a discussion of the findings. The discussion section may also include implications of the results for clinical practice.

Presenting the Content

Introductions to articles are customarily brief and concise. In addition to presenting the problem creating the need for the study, they give the purpose of the research and reasons why the author considers the study important enough to report.

The literature review may be written as part of the introductory material, especially in journals that try to keep articles short. In other instances, this review may be reported in a separate section or in a section entitled "Theoretical Framework." In any event, the literature review should be brief and specifically related to the study's purpose, hypothesis, or method, as the case may be. In a short research report one cannot report on all of the references read as part of the literature search; only the most relevant or pertinent material can be selected. Mainly, the reader will be interested in knowing that the writer is familiar with and has related his work to the major work in the field. The journal's style will be helpful here. Make note of the nature of the literature review in the articles published over a period of several months and follow that style.

If an extensive review of the work done in a special field is indeed pertinent, a review article may be in order. An article that reports on significant research in a special field, with an analysis of its contribution to the development of science or to the field under study, which also points out future research needs, can make a most important addition to the health field. There is a need for good, analytical review articles to bring together research efforts to promote the application of research findings to health care, as well as to provide direction for future investigations. A good review article is worth its weight in gold, but it is difficult to write because it involves an in-depth review of the literature and critical analysis of the research reviewed.

But, to return to the general research report, the description of the study method and of the study sample should be clearly and concisely written. Although brevity is again important, adequacy and logical presentation are perhaps even more so. The reader needs a clear and accurate description of what was done, the type of sample chosen, as well as why and how it was chosen, and the study method or procedures followed. If human subjects made up the sample, a description of how ethical standards were maintained is included here.

An outline for this section may assist the novice writer to present his material logically. For example, step-by-step or chronological order may be chosen to present the method used, or the material may be organized around the different instruments, their selection or development, and their use in the study. However the methodology section is organized, remember that it is most important for the reader to have as clear an understanding of this aspect of the research as possible to understand and evaluate the results, or, if he wishes, to replicate the study.

The analysis of the data should be presented clearly and the significance of the findings noted and discussed. Data which do not reach statistical significance should not be discussed as if they were significant. For example, authors will sometimes report that the findings were not significant and then go on to discuss the implications of the findings as if they were highly significant. This is not an acceptable practice.

In many reports of health care research, clinical significance may be as important to comment on as statistical significance. Data may be statistically significant but have little clinical significance, at least until further research is done. On the other hand, a handful of case studies of individuals with a sample too small to lend itself to statistical analysis, or even one case study of a specific group, may, if based upon careful, validated investigation, offer findings of considerable clinical significance.

Discussion of the findings and comment on their implications for health care is a most important section of the research report. Here, the study findings may be related to those studies noted earlier in the literature review. The author can compare his findings with the work of others and show how his differs from or builds upon past research. It is in this section that the author also may inject his own observations or opinions about his research and its implications, as long as he clearly notes when he is expressing his own ideas.

It is also in this section that limitations in the study, its methodology, or its results, should be noted and discussed. In fact, a discussion of the research method used and its usefulness for this type of research is an essential part of the discussion. Equally essential here is a discussion of the method of data collection and analysis and their usefulness in future research.

Finally, if there are implications for clinical practice, these should be presented. These implications may include the opinion or judgment of the investigator, but should have a relationship to the findings. And, again, if the findings were not significant, the writer should not draw conclusions or consider implications for practice based upon them as if they were significant. However, positive and negative findings relevant to health care should be discussed because of their importance to both professional practitioners and the teachers of practitioners.

Much of what has been said in this chapter relates to the most common form used in reporting research. The novice writer is urged to become familiar with the editorial style of the journal for which he is writing and to follow this style, using modifications only as they enhance his report and his personal style of writing. As he becomes a more proficient writer, he will no doubt exercise more freedom in style variations of article formats.

CHAPTER 13: The Style of the Research Report

Scholarly articles reporting on scientific investigations need not be dull and monotonous, but they can be, and too often are. Editors of professional journals and their readers agree that much of the research literature is not well written. Why? Why is the writing monotonous and hard to read when the reason for publishing an article is to have it read and understood by those who want or need the information? Perhaps one reason is that good researchers are not necessarily good writers. In any event, when research manuscripts, and even the published articles, are difficult to read and hence to interpret, this may be because too little attention has been given to the writing style, to correct sentence structure, and to logical presentation of ideas, and because the manuscript was not carefully re-read and revised by the author.

Articles written for a general audience probably will not be read at all if the reader is not attracted by the style and readability. The subject must be interesting, of course, but even if the topic attracts the reader, he will not stay with it if the content is not well stated. In professional journals, reader attention depends upon these factors as much as it does in those journals written in a more popular vein.

Although poorly written research reports may be read by those hardy souls who are truly interested in the research, such articles will have a very limited audience. And, because the writing is vague or unduly difficult to read, those who do read may make incorrect interpretations. Today's editors of professional journals are looking for reports that their readers will find interesting and that are at least moderately easy to read.

You can be more certain that you are communicating accurately if your writing is clear and straightforward and your choice of words precise. Good writing is rarely dashed off at one sitting. Most authorities agree that good writing involves rewriting. This is particularly true when writing a research report. You will need to re-read and rewrite each part of the article until you are sure that your meaning is clear.

Editorial Style and Guidelines

Editorial style is usually dictated by the periodical's requirements. As noted earlier, most journals in the health field have style guidelines for prospective authors. These guides include: the usual length of manuscripts to be submitted, the form in which it is to be submitted, and the use of illustrations, tables and figures, abbreviations, footnotes, and citation of references. Modifications which reflect the author's style may be acceptable but often only within the general framework of the journal guidelines.

Research journals rarely pay for articles but if they do, they usually indicate this in the guidelines. On the other hand, they may even charge a fee, for example for including illustrations or tables or for the number of pages used. This will also be mentioned.

As stated previously, most journal guidelines indicate the desirable length of manuscripts. If your article is longer than that recommended, careful editing to delete unnecessary content should be done before you send it in. If you put the manuscript aside for a period of time and then go back to it, it is often easier to see where material can be cut without changing the meaning of the paper. Most of us use far more words than we need and there is plenty of room for pruning! But do not despair if you find such cutting difficult. Most authors have trouble deleting material from their articles.

If, after editing your research report, it is still too long, perhaps it lends itself to a two-part article or to two completely different articles. Most journals do not encourage two-part articles but some will occasionally consider them. If the length of the proposed article is only slightly longer than recommended and it seems impossible to shorten it further, perhaps the best course is to submit it as is and let the editor decide whether it can be published without cutting.

Going back to your paper after a lapse of time also provides an opportunity to check your style and whether your meaning is clear throughout. Reading the paper aloud is a good way to do this. If a part of it does not read smoothly, you'll know that it needs special attention.

Another method of checking your manuscript for style and clarity is to ask someone else to read the paper for you. This approach should be taken only after you have done as much rewriting as you feel you can. This reader should be someone you trust to be an honest critic and to help you locate where meaning is unclear or style cumbersome or monotonous.

Title and Headings

Titles of articles reporting on research should be descriptive of the content and not "cute" or "catchy." Catchy titles may be quite appropriate for popular journals but not for research journals. Readers of research journals are particularly interested in knowing what the article is about and look to the title for this information. Also, titles are used by indexers as clues to headings under which to include the article. In addition to being factual, the title should be as brief as is consistent with its informational purpose.

In addition to the title, subject headings are important guides for the prospective reader. He can scan the article quickly and by means of the headings obtain an overall idea of the nature of the content. Furthermore, as he reads the article, the headings, like road signs, help guide him through the content. If you have used an outline to prepare the article, this outline may provide you with the headings you need.

Subheadings may be used for articles that are long or require subdivisions in addition to major headings. For example, the section on methodology may need subheads under which the various instruments used for data collection are described.

Tables and Figures

Tables and figures are often important to the research report and are indicated when the data can be expressed better in this form than in the narrative. Most journals recommend that their use be limited since space is at a premium and illustrations are costly.

Tables should be carefully done and checked for accuracy. Like article titles, titles of tables should state precisely what is in them. Figures, including charts and graphs, should be accurate and prepared on a good grade of white paper using black India ink. Chart and graph are frequently used interchangeably. A chart presents data or information in methodical, tabulated form or in graphic form: a graph may take the form of either a bar or line graph. It is a good idea to accompany graphs or charts with the data on which they are based. These data are not for publication but are useful to the editor if the chart or graph needs to be redrawn or the data cannot be clearly interpreted from it. If you plan to use pictures, they should be good quality, black and white glossy prints unless the journal uses color, in which case you may submit color photographs.

In planning illustrations, simplicity is desirable whenever possible. Complex tables or graphs are not only difficult for the reader to interpret but, if they are long, may pose problems in reducing them to fit the page. And remember, although a good illustration may be better than a thousand words, an illustration which is repetitious of a description already in the text, or one which can be more easily described in the narrative, is superfluous.

Abbreviations

Acronyms abound in today's world and are found in all forms of writing. Spell out the acronym the first time it is used; for example, "American Medical Association

(AMA)" even though it seems to be familiar to everyone in the health field. This procedure will keep the reader on the right track.

In research literature many special abbreviations and symbols are used and it is of the utmost importance to be accurate, especially when abbreviating drugs, weights, and measures, as well as various physical conditions, for example, ventricular septal defect (VSD). Greek letters used as statistical symbols should be spelled out in the margins of the paper if they are drawn in and could possibly be misinterpreted. Care should also be taken to insure accuracy of chemical symbols and formulae.

Generally the excessive use of abbreviations that are not standard slows the reader by making it necessary for him to constantly remind himself what they mean.

References and Footnotes

Research journals each have their style for references and footnotes. Some journals place only general footnotes on the same page as the content to which it refers and all references at the end of the article. Others list both general footnotes and references in the same place.

In preparing the manuscript, remember that the journal's guidelines for prospective authors almost always indicate the style of references and footnotes to use and give examples. Further examples, can, of course, be found in any issue of the journal you have selected for your article.

If you keep reference cards that are complete and accurate, you will have no difficulty adapting your references to the style suggested. Keeping complete references of all work cited cannot be overemphasized. When incomplete or inaccurate citations are made in a manuscript and you have not kept reference cards, you may need to take much additional time and effort to go back and relocate them to make the necessary corrections. Sometimes a valuable reference may even have to be deleted simply because you neglected to keep a complete record and you are unable to relocate it.

The Author's Personal Style

Much about an author's personal style is already covered in Part One and will not be repeated here. However, there are a few things that may be said about writing the research report. As mentioned at the beginning of this chapter, research articles need not be dull and monotonous; however, because of the nature of the content, special care needs to be taken if you want to have an interesting, well written article.

Voice

A common problem of authors of research manuscripts is the frequent use of the passive voice when a more lively narrative and greater ease of reading would be promoted by the more liberal use of the active voice. This tendency to use the passive voice may be an attempt to be impersonal and thus more objective, but unfortunately it results in cumbersome, pedantic writing and sometimes even a lack of clarity.

The following paragraph is quoted first in its original form, using the active voice and flowing smoothly, then its content is transposed into the passive voice. The difference in reader impact is clear.

The Behavioral Checklist. This checklist, [was] devised by the authors and . . ., is an observational tool completed by a rater. It lists the ten component parts of dependence and independence denoted by Beller and gives examples of behavior under each component that may be observed by the nurse in caring for a hospitalized adult patient. Dependence subscales are: . . . . Independence subscales are: . . . . The rater lists the frequency the behavior is exhibited within a given time period. In this study, the authors were the raters. To gather behavioral checklist data, they spent two hours in the morning giving care and helping with breakfast.*

Written in the passive voice, this paragraph might read:

The Behavioral Checklist. This checklist was devised by the authors and . . ., is an observational tool which was to be completed by the rater. Beller's ten component parts of dependence and independence were listed and examples of behavior were given under each component that could be observed by the nurse in caring for a hospitalized patient. The dependence subscales were listed as: . . . . Independence subscales were listed as: . . . . Within a given time period the frequency of the behavior exhibited was listed by the raters who were the authors. Two hours were spent by them in the morning giving care and helping with breakfast so that the data on patient behavior on the checklist could be gathered.

Although the above is not an extreme example, It illustrates writing entirely in the passive voice. The following is another example showing how information given in the passive voice can even become misleading.

Because information gain is only one desirable goal of the course unit on drug addiction, also measured were possible attitude changes in the two groups relating to instructional television and how the subjects' perception of experiences related to various aspects of the course are influenced by this media.

The above is what sometimes happens when the passive voice is used and the writer tries to get too much into

---

*Derdiarian A, Clough D: Patients' dependence and independence levels on the prehospitalization-postdischarge continuum, Nurs Res 25:29, Jan.-Feb. 1976. Copyright © February 1976, the American Journal of Nursing Company. Quoted with permission from *Nursing Research.*

one sentence. For example, widely separated subjects and verbs may not agree, as you can note in the last sentence where the singular subject, "perception," does not agree with the plural verb, "are." Also, we can be reasonably certain that the author did not mean that attitude measurement was "because information gain was only one desirable goal." More simply stated the paragraph might read:

> Information gain was only one goal of the unit of study on drug addiction; attitude change was also considered an important outcome. This study examined the influence of instructional television on student attitudes toward drug addiction.

Another reason noted for the cumbersome use of the passive voice in research writing is avoiding the use of "I" or "we" (if more than one investigator is reporting). Authors of research articles tend to shy away from the use of "I" and to use "the author" instead. However, there is no reason why "I" cannot be used when it proves awkward to do otherwise. The third person, passive voice approach, such as "it is believed," is no longer considered necessary to denote objectivity.*

Paragraph Structure

Another very common way of making it difficult for the reader is poor organization of content into paragraphs. Only one major idea or theme should be included in each paragraph. This one idea is elaborated or explained in the paragraph. But repetition of the same idea several times in the same paragraph, with the mistaken idea that it clarifies or emphasizes it, frequently only slows the reader. The following is an example of this kind of circular writing:

---

*See American Psychological Association, Publication Manual of the American Psychological Association, 2nd ed., Washington, D.C., 1974, p. 28.

Table 7 reveals that respondents who were single and who were in college one year after high school graduation were more likely to complete their baccalaureate degree than were married respondents in college one year after graduation. This finding was even stronger for those who were married and had one or more children. Thus, respondents in college one year after high school graduation who were single were more likely to complete their baccalaureate degree than were married respondents and especially those married respondents who had one or more children and our second hypothesis was thus supported.

A simpler version might read:

Table 7 reveals that respondents who were single and who were in college one year after high school graduation were more likely to complete their baccalaureate degree than were married respondents in college one year after graduation. This finding was even stronger for those who were married and had one or more children. These findings supported our second hypothesis.

Common Grammatical Errors

For the most part, a report of completed research is written in the past tense since you are writing about something that has already taken place; however, there are exceptions to this and certain parts of the report are correctly written in the present tense. Thus, one may find the present tense useful when discussing the results or the implications of the findings of the study, or when commenting on the contents of a table in the report; for example, "Table 1 shows that . . . ."

A common fault of the novice author is a tendency to mix tenses. This may be avoided by going back over the manuscript and checking it carefully to insure consistency in tenses. For example, make sure that you do not start a paragraph in one tense and end it in another without a good reason for the change.

It is also good practice to check for lack of agreement between the subjects and their verbs. As illustrated previously, this lack of agreement commonly occurs when the subject is some distance from its verb and there are several plural words in between. Three words often used in research writing pose particular problems in research reporting. The nouns "data," "phenomena," and "criteria" are all plural and normally require a plural verb. One frequently sees: "the data was" or "one criteria is" when the correct form is "the data were" and "one criterion is." The singular forms are: datum, phenomenon, and criterion.

Words

Much has already been said about the use of words, and especially about the use of jargon, in the first part of this book. Emphasis here will be on the more precise use of words in research reporting and on the avoidance of words or language thought to be scholarly but which do not apply to your paper.

The careful use of words is an important goal of all writing. It becomes even more important in the research article where specificity of meaning is a primary concern. Careless use of words or abbreviations, as for example, the use of "effect" for "affect," "principle" for "principal," "mitigate" for "militate," and e.g. for i.e. should be avoided at all costs. There are other incorrect usages that I could mention, but these are ones recently observed in the literature and frequently found in manuscripts submitted for publication.

As to the use of scientific jargon, certain words and phrases seem to be the fashion of the times. They are overused for a period of time and then go out of style. One tendency that seems to be constant in the use of jargon, however, is the use of invented words, particularly verbs dressed up as nouns, or nouns made into verbs or adjectives. These have little or no place in research literature. Three examples seen in recent research articles are: operationalize, prioritize, and answerability. A cursory review of the literature would turn up many more. You might find it interesting to keep a list of those you find in order to remind yourself not to use them.

Some writers tend to use obscure or complex phrases which they consider scholarly even though the meaning would be much clearer if simpler language were used. One example comes to mind: the use of "cognitive consistency" meaning to "think alike" or to "have similar attitudes." The following is a short piece written to show the effect of the use of scholarly jargon. We are all familiar with the beauty of the original.

Professor Hamlet's Soliloquy

("To Be or Not To Be" translated into Educational Jargon)

> To maintain this bio-chemical entity or
> to terminate this unit of personnel,
> *that* is the focal point of this on-going
> problem-solving process.
>
> Whether by some value system
> one may arrive at the policy determination
> that random socio-psychological stress
> may be tolerated, or to initiate purposive
> acting-out to re-structure the situation?
>
> To terminate, to hibernate, there's the
> pertinent decision-making emergent from
> our fact-finding, for even in the passive state
> what fantasy formation may eventuate?
>
> Aye, there's the rub!

Few of us aspire to be another Shakespeare but by using simple, clearly stated sentences, cohesive paragraphs, and, for the most part, the active voice, our research reports may turn out to be pleasantly readable, or at least straightforward and easily understood prose.

---

*Amrine M: Professor Hamlet's Soliloquy, *Phi Delta Kappan* 39:May 1958. Quoted with permission of *Phi Delta Kappan*.

CHAPTER 14: The Abstract

When you submit a research article to a journal, you are required also to submit a special form of summary, called an abstract, of the article. It is customary for journals carrying research literature to print the abstract at the head of the article. These are commonly known as journal abstracts and serve two purposes: To indicate to prospective readers the gist of the article and to be used by journals that publish only abstracts, as for example, *Pyschological Abstracts* or *Excerpta Medica.*

Writing the Abstract

In a letter written over 300 years ago, Pascal commented, "I have made this letter longer than usual because I lack the time to make it shorter."* You may find it difficult to write an abstract, especially an informative one, in 100 to 200 words, but with a bit of rewriting and condensing, it can be done.

The journal's guidelines will very likely give you some directions as to the length of the abstract and may indicate the type they want. If not, examples are readily available in various issues of the journal you have selected.

A good method to keep in mind in writing the abstract is to follow your outline. Begin with a statement of the problem or the purpose and follow this with a sentence or two about the methodology (including the sample used), the data analysis, and the findings. These cannot be discussed in any detail so only the most significant facts should be given. There is no need to include the literature review or any other background. However, if a particular theory served as a framework for the study, you may wish to mention it. In any event, keep to a brief,

---

*Blaise Pascal (1623-1662), Provincial Letters XVI (written sometime after 1656).

factual description of the content of the article. If you are abstracting someone else's article, avoid evaluations of the report; these are not appropriate in an abstract.

After writing the abstract, try to condense it further by deleting adjectives, adverbs, or phrases that do not really enhance the meaning of a sentence or add to the reader's knowledge about the study which follows. And remember, do not put into the abstract anything not appearing in the article and do not use quotations from the article.

As with any other form of writing, practice will improve your abstracting skill and style. Brief and concise, but accurate and informative abstracts are invaluable tools for the researcher. Not only will your abstract assist the journal reader, but the researcher looking for studies in his field is dependent upon it to pinpoint his selection of articles from the myriad available in the general subject area. Also, persons in the particular field of interest often read abstracts as a means of current awareness of new knowledge.

One last word, authors vary considerably in their style of writing abstracts. An abstract can include all of the necessary points of interest to the researcher-reader and still not be interestingly written. As noted in Chapter 3 under "Personal Style," straightforward writing and a logical format will help you to attain a pleasing, readable style.

The following is an example of an informative abstract:*

A concept attainment model of diagnosis was used to study the influence of inferential ability and restricted-unrestricted information conditions on 60 nurses'

---

*Gordon M: Predictive strategies in diagnostic tasks. Nurs Res 29:39, Jan-Feb. 1980. Copyright © 1980. The American Journal of Nursing Company. Quoted with permission from *Nursing Research.*

hypothesis-scanning strategies, diagnostic accuracy, and confidence in two diagnostic tasks. A selection paradigm, similar to the game of Twenty Questions, was employed, and it was assumed that verbal reports of how information was being utilized were reliable indicators of scanning procedures. Analysis of variance, t tests, chi-square analyses, and the Cochrane Q test were used in data analyses. Subjects' behavior approximated a model strategy of predictive hypothesis testing in diagnostic concept attainment tasks involving surgical complications. Neither the interaction between inferential ability and information conditions nor the effect of inferential ability alone influenced the dependent variables, although prolonged predictive hypothesis testing and unrestricted information conditions were associated with greater inaccuracies. Implications for nursing history taking and diagnosis are discussed.

In less than 150 words the abstract gives the essential information contained in the article.

Types of Abstracts

The usual form of abstract which the beginning researcher needs to master is the type cited above, the informative. However, there are several other types and it is useful to understand the distinctions.

Taylor identifies six types of abstracts according to the nature of their content.* The simplest are: those classified by title only; those composed of key sentences generated from the article by computer (the autoabstract); and the "slanted abstract" which extracts only that material of special interest to a particular discipline. The "title only" abstract appears in abstract journals and provides only the bibliographic information about the article and then

---

*Taylor SD: How to prepare an abstract, Nurs Outlook 15:61-63, Sept. 1967.

indicates where the original abstracts may be found. This practice is used when the abstract has appeared in another abstract journal. The more usual kind of abstract falls into one of the three remaining content categories: 1) the annotative, 2) the indicative, or 3) the informative.

The journal to which you submit your article will usually specify which abstract form they use. The following guidelines may be helpful in distinguishing between the three most common:

The Annotative Abstract. The simplest form of abstract is the annotated one. It is the briefest and in a few lines gives the reader an idea of the nature of the content of the article. It is really an explanatory note indicating the major purpose or theme of the article.

The Indicative Abstract. Slightly more information about the article is given in an indicative abstract than can be found in the annotated one. It is usually a few lines longer and includes a brief description of the article's content. It provides rather general information amplifying the title.

The Informative Abstract. Where the purpose is to communicate to the reader as complete a summary as possible within the abstract format, the informative type of abstract is indicated. To include more information, of course, the abstract may need to be a bit longer than the annotated or the indicative types, but it is usually limited to 100 to 200 words. Many readers prefer this type because it gives them the gist of the article and thus helps them more readily decide about reading further. Also, when published in an abstract journal, it tells them enough to decide whether they wish to go back to the original article.

Many readers use this type of abstract as an easy method of keeping abreast of a growing body of literature. Therefore, readers should be knowledgeable about the derivation of the abstracts they use. In some cases abstracts in abstract journals are not written by the author. For example, in addition to the journal abstracts, other abstracts may be written by subject experts, by professional abstracters, or rewritten by a non-author for a special purpose. Subject experts may be volunteer abstracters and their name may appear at the end of the abstract.

CHAPTER 15: Editorial Evaluation

Editorial decision about a manuscript is given only after expert evaluation of both the manuscript and the research reported in it. The purpose of editorial review is to select and publish well-written reports that meet the standards set by scientists in the field. Thus, because of the expert screening, publication in a professional journal implies that the research reported meets an acceptable standard of quality.

The System of Evaluation

To achieve the needed expert evaluation, professional journals carrying research articles make use of peer groups, such as editorial boards or referees. These board members or referees are experts in the various fields of research in which the journal is interested. They serve in a volunteer capacity, considering this activity to be one of their professional responsibilities. Their names usually appear in the journal, sometimes on the masthead page. They are expected to review manuscripts in their special field of expertise and supply the editor with their critique of the research and recommendations about acceptance, rejection, or revision of the manuscript. To insure as much freedom from bias as possible, some journals send "anonymous" manuscripts to the referees, that is, the name of the author does not appear on it.

Referees are expected to complete their evaluations within a reasonable time, for example, in four to six weeks. Each manuscript is usually sent to two or three referees although, if necessary, additional expert opinion may be sought, especially when the original referees do not agree.

The Nature of the Evaluation

The first evaluation of the manuscript is made by the journal editor for the purpose of general disposition of the paper. The editor may reject certain manuscripts outright without the use of referees — these are the papers that obviously do not come within the purpose of the journal. Those that do meet the objectives or purpose of the journal are then sent to appropriate referees, selected on the basis of their interests and expertise in given areas.

Most journals using referees have a form to be completed by the referees and returned to the editor with the manuscript. These forms are rather simple and include the title of the manuscript, a place to check whether it is acceptable, not acceptable, or acceptable with reservations (with revision), and space for a critique. If revisions are indicated, the referee is expected to indicate what these should be and why.

Some of the areas to be scrutinized by the referees are:

Purpose of the Research. Is this stated and clearly related to the reported investigation?

Review of the Literature. Is the review concise and relevant? Does it include all references that have special relevance to the research, thus indicating that the investigator was knowledgeable about the most important studies in the field?

The Research Itself. Is the design appropriate to the kind of problem under investigation? Was the sample adequate and appropriate? Were the rights of individuals protected? Were instruments for data collection appropriate and were their validity and reliability reported? Were the right statistics used and the data analysis and findings reported objectively? If generalizations were made, were these in line with the findings or did the investigator overgeneralize? Does the research add anything new to the research literature?

The Manuscript Itself. Is the manuscript well organized, clearly written, and concise without being superficial?

The above does not represent all that is examined in a research paper, but will give you some idea of the kinds of judgments made. The nature of the critique will depend somewhat upon the type of research done. For example, different kinds of things will be examined in a paper reporting on historical research than in one reporting on experimental clinical research.

The Decision Process

The referees' reviews are then evaluated by the editor who makes the final decision about publication. Several factors influence this decision: 1) the reviews from referees; 2) relative merits of all the manuscripts available for publication; and 3) the available journal space.

The referees' reviews carry considerable weight in the editor's own evaluation and decision. However, most editors of research journals, like editors of other professional journals, receive many more manuscripts than they can publish. A large number of those rejected are clearly not acceptable, others may be borderline and rejected only because they have to compete with much better manuscripts. Even some of the better ones may have to be rejected because space is not available. If space is limited, then the editor must carefully evaluate the relative merits or contributions of the manuscripts and select those of most value for the readers. Journals that charge authors for publication, usually by the page, may have more freedom to add extra pages to accommodate additional articles, although it may be necessary to set limits even under these circumstances.

Reasons for Rejection

Some of the most common reasons for manuscript rejection are: 1) the author's ignorance of the journal's purpose, the type of articles published, and the format and style used; 2) poor organization and lack of clarity which result in a paper that is difficult to evaluate because it is hard to interpret; 3) superficial treatment of the content; 4) careless citing of references; 5) the paper adds nothing new to the literature in the field; and 6) the quality of the research reported does not meet acceptable standards.*

Sometimes the novice writer whose first effort is rejected can learn a great deal. Some editors will send comments that are indeed helpful in planning the next paper or in re-working the rejected manuscript. If no comments are returned with the rejected manuscript you may write and ask for them. The comments may not always be forthcoming, but you do increase your chances of learning what was wrong. If no comments are sent as a result of your letter, go over your manuscript and compare it with those published in the journal to see if you can discover for yourself how and why your paper differed. Or, you might ask someone who has published to critique your paper for you. Learn as much as you can from your rejection so that future efforts will be more likely to be successful — don't let rejections stop you. Sometimes a rewritten paper gets published in another type of publication more appropriate to the content.

Working with the Editor

By now you have some idea of what editors are and what they do. They carry ultimate responsibility for the quality of the journal they edit. They seek the very best manuscripts reporting significant and well-designed research. They try to be one step ahead of the times and so also look for manuscripts reporting research they believe has important implications for the future. They answer your query letters about your prospective manuscript, they work with referees, and they make final decisions on manuscripts.

---

*See Archer JD: Attributes of a rejected manuscript, JAMA 232(2):165, April 14, 1975.

Additionally they edit manuscripts which have been accepted, checking data for accuracy; rephrasing when ideas are not well expressed, and making other minor revisions; checking references or seeing that this is done; and in general, getting the manuscript ready for publication. Finally, the edited manuscripts are sent to the authors for approval prior to publication.

As mentioned earlier, manuscripts may be accepted with recommendations for revision. When this happens, the editor will send the author suggestions — his own as well as those of the referees. If you receive an acceptance qualified in this way, do not be discouraged. After your initial disappointment, go over your paper carefully and attempt to see the reasoning behind the suggestions offered. If you have questions, call or write the editor. If they have made suggestions for revisions, it means that they have more than a passing interest in your paper.

When you are satisfied that you understand the reasons for the suggestions, begin revising the paper. You may find that rewriting is hard work — we do resist changing our own writing — but the effort is usually worth it. Stick with it and, when your have completed the revision, try it out once more on someone who can evaluate it for you. Then send it back to the editor as soon as possible.

In some instances revisions go through the same process of referee evaluation as did the original copy; in other instances, the editor may make the final decision based upon the quality of your revision.

Working with an editor on a revision or on the editing of an accepted manuscript can be challenging and, at the same time, a learning experience in perfecting your written expression. Much of the learning will come from making the suggested changes or in noting the editing done; the challenge will be to use the editorial suggestions to enhance your paper and ultimately insure its publication.

Finally, when your accepted manuscript has been edited and sent to you for your approval, go over it carefully. Make sure that any revisions accurately reflect your meaning. Also, make any corrections that you find necessary; however, additions or deletions to the manuscript should be kept to a minimum unless the editor has suggested them.

CHAPTER 16: The Research Grant Proposal

Considerable preparation and planning are essential to the writing of a research grant proposal. A grant proposal is written with a specific granting agency in mind; therefore, there must be a clearly identifiable relationship between the research or project proposed and the purpose or interests of the granting agency. It is important to find out as much as you can about the agency's program, its special interests, and the general form in which proposals should be submitted. Make certain that your research is within the scope of the agency's interest.

Many granting agencies, particularly the federal ones, have special forms to be completed and guidelines to use in writing the proposal. Foundations may simply ask for a letter explaining your proposal, but you will find that it is still a good idea to follow a format similar to that requested by the federal agencies.

When you plan to approach a federal agency, obtain the necessary materials far enough in advance to be able to study them thoroughly before developing your proposal. It is wise to follow the form suggested; however, some slight modifications occasionally can be justified if your research or project design does not lend itself to the type of description required. For example, the form may be geared to experimental research but your project involves the development and evaluation of a new community health service for a particular segment of the community. If your description is justified by the type of study design, the modifications likely will be acceptable.

A grant proposal or application is a logical presentation of what you plan to do, how you plan to go about it, and why you think the study is important. The relationship of the various parts of the proposal needs to be identified and logically presented. In general, the application includes the following sections: the problem to be studied; the objectives of the research; the literature review; the methodology, including data analysis and a timetable of activities; facilities and resources; and a suggested budget. If the proposal is for a special project, plans for the evaluation will be required as part of the method. An abstract of the proposal is usually also requested.

As with all professional writing, the grant proposal should be written in a straightforward, lucid style.

The Problem to be Studied

A clear statement of the problem which prompted the study, or the hypothesis to be tested, will get you off to a good start. This statement should indicate the nature of the problem and the reasons why the problem needs to be studied, or why a new approach to solving the problem, the one you propose, is needed. The reviewers who will make the decision about your proposal will be particularly interested in the significance of the problem and must be convinced that a study is needed to solve it. Your justification of this significance will help them understand it and, therefore, should be in sufficient detail to provide for their full understanding of why you feel this particular piece of research is important.

If exploratory or pilot studies have been made, include a statement about these in the discussions of the study's significance. Reports of this preliminary work should be added to the application as part of the appendix. These reports, together with your understanding of the problem and the need for the research, will assist in establishing your competence in the area.

The Objectives

This section may be relatively brief but all of the objectives specific to your project should be listed. You might start with a statement of the major or final goal of the study and then follow this with a listing of all of the specific objectives that need to be met in achieving the final goal.

Primarily a listing of objectives, this section may not need much in the way of discussion. It should logically follow the discussion of the various aspects of the problem discussed in the previous section and tie in with the design, methodology, and timetable sections.

The Literature Review

Support for the need for a particular type of research proposed is further provided by a selective review of the literature that represents the significant work done in the area. Your review should be a critical evaluation, not just a description, of the literature. Additionally, indicate how you plan to build on or add to prior research. If you believe prior research has used inappropriate approaches, discuss why you think these were inappropriate and why you feel your own approach may prove to be more effective. If you plan to build on the research of others, explain why this is indicated and how your approach will do this. Finally, if you wish to replicate another study, be sure to indicate why replication seems the thing to do, for example, the importance of testing the original study on a different kind of sample or on a larger, more representative sample.

Keep the literature review relatively brief. It is not necessary to report on all you have read but do report the important studies that have a bearing on your research. The granting agency needs to know that you are familiar with the significant work in the study area, are well grounded in the theory or theories involved, and are therefore competent to do the study for which you are seeking funds. If you have any question about including something you have read, err on the side of discussing it. It is better to include a bit more than you need than to leave out something important.

If your study is based on a particular theory or theories, a discussion of the literature regarding the theory is imperative, as is a clear indication of the relationship of the theory to your own study.

123

In summary, a brief but comprehensive presentation of the literature of significance to your study and providing a rationale for it, will assist the reviewers in evaluating both the need for the study and your own background of understanding for carrying it out.

The Research Method

In presenting the methodology you have planned, it might be helpful to set up your timetable first. Although in your application the timetable will follow the discussion of methodology, setting it down first may help you to develop the methodology section in a more logical order — and it must be emphasized that logical order is very important here.

Before you start writing a research grant proposal, the methodology you plan to use and the steps you plan to take to accomplish the study should be so carefully thought through that there is no problem in describing them logically. In describing your methods, include their limitations as well as their strengths.

If instruments have been developed, explain them and place illustrations of them in the appendix. Show how the instruments will gather the data you are seeking, how appropriate they are to the research, and how you plan to use them. Indicate their reliability and validity, or how they will be tested. If the instruments have not yet been developed, give the reasons why and show how you plan to develop and test them.

When describing the expected data and subsequent analysis, include any specific statistical analyses you plan to use, when this is indicated, and give a brief explanation of why you are using them. It is a good idea to have a statistician check the type of data analyses for you. According to Gortner, all too often data analysis plans are not specified or are described insufficiently to indicate that the investigator knows what kind of data he will have and how they will be analyzed.*

Finally, because of the importance of the rights and welfare of human subjects, a plan to protect these rights is an integral part of any research where humans are involved. In your proposal include your methods of obtaining informed consent, and of providing for rights to privacy, confidentiality of data, and protection against physical or psychological harm.

Since this section of the proposal will be most carefully scrutinized, it must be logically and completely presented. Reviewers will be looking for assurance of your knowledge of the problem and of the research procedure. Vagueness and lack of detail will indicate that you have not adequately thought through the problem and the rationale for the steps in the procedure. Reviewers are not looking for a long drawn out description but they do need to see the project as a whole and to identify the essential details of the procedure you plan to follow.

Your timetable should follow the methodology section or serve as the final part of that section. A carefully set up timetable does two things: it gives the granting agency the necessary overview of the research; and it provides a means of estimating the time required to complete the research. If you are asking for a three-year grant and the timetable shows that you may need a two- or three-year extension of the grant, explain the reasons for the additional years and how you plan to manage them. Some agencies will grant an extension of funds if they are pleased with the progress made in the first part of the work. However, it may be wise to plan your research in two parts so that the first part is fairly complete in itself in the event an extension is not forthcoming.

---

*Gortner SR, Research grants: what they are not and should be. Nurs Res 20:294, July-Aug. 1971.

Resources and Facilities

Your proposal should indicate clearly the personnel you expect to work on the research. The research or project director and the principal investigator may be one and the same; on the other hand, the principal investigator may be the person in the institution seeking a grant who assumes ultimate responsibility but delegates direction of the research to a competent researcher. In addition, list all other personnel, both full time and part time, such as research associates, assistants, and secretaries. For those already selected, resumés should be included in an appendix. If the use of consultants is planned, the type of consultants can be indicated and their names given if they have already agreed to serve. In the latter instance, their education and experience should also be included in the appendix.

All facilities available for use in the study, such as office space, computers, or other equipment should be noted.

The Budget

Most granting agencies provide guidelines and a form for presentation of the anticipated budget. The usual expenses incurred in doing a study will be included, such as personnel salaries and benefits, consultant fees, equipment, supplies, telephone, and travel costs. If there are patient costs, these are included and there is usually additional space for "other" expenses. When the proposal is for more than one year, the budget is itemized for each year. Budgeted expenses should be in line with the actual anticipated costs characteristic of the locality where the project is planned.

Often, some items such as office space are contributed to the project. This may be noted in the general statement of the proposal.

The Abstract

Most granting agencies require an abstract or summary of the study to accompany the grant application. A form is supplied for this purpose. Keep the abstract brief but include all important factors. The abstracts are used by the governmental agencies and some of the private foundations to submit to the Smithsonian Science Information Exchange in Washington, D.C., an agency that supplies information about on-going research to interested investigators.

It is perhaps the last page of the application you complete but the abstract is the first one read by the granting agency's review panel. Therefore, it must present a succinct statement of the purpose, objectives, the study procedure, the amount of money requested, and of your qualifications for the proposed project. Granting agencies often use the summary to screen applications to determine which meet their criteria and whether the project procedure is sound and logical. Your summary, therefore, must be carefully written in order to present an accurate overview of the proposal. It cannot be hastily thrown together after you have completed your application or the result may be a good application overlooked because of a poor abstract.

Grantsmanship

Much has been said about "grantsmanship" and the importance of writing good proposals. It should be emphasized here that good proposals involve at least two things: a significant research idea and a clear, logical presentation of the project proposal. If you are writing your first proposal, make sure you have a significant research idea. This means a genuine problem and a logical procedure, with an appropriate data analysis plan. Then, if possible, get some expert help with the writing. Do the initial writing yourself but ask someone who has had experience to go over it and make certain it does justice to your project. The Foundation Center, 888 Seventh Avenue, New York, N.Y. 10106, can provide you with information about funding sources. Its libraries, located in various parts of the country, contain a wealth of resources on foundations and on proposal writing.

In general, reviewers will:

. . . consider the specific research plan proposed, the scientific, social, medical, or health service significance of the topic under study, the state of knowledge in that field, the feasibility of the research, the competence and dedication to the project of the principal investigator and of his supporting staff, the adequacy of the facilities available to him, the potential usefulness, generalizability, or heuristic value of the results, and the appropriateness of the proposed budget for the work outlined.*

Some General Comments

You may have read all that has been written about writing the research article or grant proposal, but you still must take that first step and begin putting your ideas on paper.

For some, the first article is the hardest; for others, the words flow easily. However, in writing research reports, unusual care should be taken that the reporting is accurate — accurate in the use of words and accurate as to the reporting of the research.

Why is accuracy so important? Why, of course, you will say, because other researchers depend upon the truth of what you write and you want it to be so clear and accurate that there will be no misinterpretation. Also, research

---

*U.S. Department of Health, Education and Welfare, Public Health Service, National Institutes of Health, Division of Research Grants, Information for National Institutes of Health Research Grant Applicants. Washington, DC.

articles become part of the archival material of the profession. They remain as landmarks and are used as reference points long after they are reported — even those findings that have been disputed or disproven.

Do not let the archival nature of research articles frighten you or deter your interest in writing. As stated earlier, your research is not complete until it is reported in the literature. And remember, all researchers had to start with that first report!

Remember to keep the title short and specific to the research reported. Give a thought to the number of authors listed. It is best to keep these to the minimum who really helped with the report. If others need to be recognized, do this in a footnote or in an acknowledgement section at the end of your report. One to three authors seems to be adequate for most articles. An article with more than five authors raises questions about the nature and value of each author's contribution to the article.

And finally, keep in mind a few of the suggestions made to help you along the way. Good writing means careful rewriting, whether it be writing in a lighter vein as discussed in Part One or research writing. Your first article may need to be reworked several times. Just put it aside, then come back to it periodically. When near completion, have a good critic look it over for you. And when you feel you have done your best, send it off. Let's hope your first attempt will be successful!

APPENDIX A
TRANSITIONAL WORDS, PHRASES, SENTENCES*

To Show Sequence:
First, Second, Third
Primarily
Logically
Chronologically

To Show Consequence:
Therefore
Consequently
As a result
For this reason
Accordingly

To Show Comparison:
In the same manner
Similarly
In the same way
By comparison

To Show Contrast:
By contrast
Yet
On the other hand
Instead
On the contrary

To Illustrate:
For example
For instance
Take the case of
To illustrate

To Show Time-Relationship:
Next
Later on
Then
Moments later
A year later
The next day
At present
Meanwhile
Earlier
At the same time

To Make Additions:
Moreover
Furthermore
Also
Besides
In addition

To Sum Up:
In conclusion
In sum
Finally
In other words
In short
To summarize

Transitional Sentence:
Here is the reason we favor
this procedure:

---

*Reproduced from Editor's Manual of Editorial, Production and Publishing Procedures, American Journal of Nursing Company, with permission of the author, Professor Julian Elfenbien.

Transitional Paragraph:

We have been discussing methods of getting cohesiveness in our writing. Let us turn now to methods and techniques used to tie together our sequences of thought.

APPENDIX B
WRITER'S CHECKLIST

Now that you have several pages written on your project, go over it with the following questions in mind:

1. What message are you trying to convey? Check your lead paragraph. If it doesn't tell the reader your main idea or purpose, rewrite it.

2. Is your material organized? Does it flow smoothly? Did you follow your outline? Are your points well developed? Have you used transitional phrases to help the reader along?

3. Have you kept your readers in mind? Will they understand and appreciate your message? If you've described how to do something, can your readers do it?

4. Have you documented, footnoted, or referenced the material where necessary? If the project has been accepted for publication, have you obtained written permission(s) for direct quotes of more than 200 words, or tables, graphs, charts, and illustrations?

5. Have you checked your spelling, particularly proper names?

6. Have you checked tenses, punctuation, and grammar? Have you conducted a careful "which" hunt?

7. Have you kept your language *simple,* and avoided clichés, jargon, cuteness, and other pitfalls?

8. Does your manuscript lead to a logical conclusion and not leave your reader hanging?

9. Have you made a copy for your own files?

APPENDIX C

JARGONESE, COLORLESS VERBS, AND GLAMOR TERMS
(With tongue in cheek)

Jargonese

Conceptual model — diagramming an idea

Conceptual framework — more of the same

Crisis intervention — doing something about the mess

Utilize — use

Behavioral objectives — what you're expected to do

Cognitive objective — why you're doing it

Paradigm — model

Frame of reference — where we're at

Ombudsman — the patients' friend and advocate

Patients' advocate — ombudsman

Logistics — how to move people or things around

Systems model — diagramming an idea systematically

Facilitator — a boss by any other name is still a boss

Glamor Words

clout — hitting base

accountability — responsibility with feeling

confrontation — letting somebody else have it

encounter group — the "in" thing

ping-ponging — "see another specialist"

impacted on — defies definition!

finalize — get it over with

eyeball to eyeball — humanly impossible

zip — nothing

Colorless Verbs

accomplished — got it done; finished it

achieved — worked hard and got somewhere

attained — arrived at

carried out — we did the experiment

conducted — did

effected — see achieved

experienced — felt it, or did it
facilitated — made it easier
given — already established
implemented — see facilitated
indicated — pointed it out
involved — drawn into the whole thing
obtained — got
occurred — happened
performed — see conducted
produced — see accomplished
required — took doing

APPENDIX D
GUIDELINES FOR CRITIQUING A MANUSCRIPT

1. Title — review it carefully — is it stuffy? Too long? Too cutesy?

   Suggest possible alternatives to editor.
   Comment on your reactions to the title.

2. Lead paragraph:

   Think! Would you continue reading this article? If not, suggest (and hunt for in the manuscript) a different lead.

   Does it tell you what you want to know about the content (who, what, and where — how and when)?

3. Is the article on a whole consistent, logical, helpful? Is it verbose (overwritten?) Is it vague? (Should the author clarify certain points?) Is it dull? (Were *you* bored?)

4. The five "C's":

   Clarity
   Completenness
   Conciseness
   Concreteness
   Comprehensiveness

5. Suggest ways to jazz up the content. Does it need anecdotes or cases to verify the *point* of the article?

6. Are the references accurate and adequate? Are they definitely related to the content?

7. Put the manuscript away for a day or so and then read it again. Do you have the same reactions?

8. Does it have proper transitional phrases (i.e., are you carried along in sequence as you read?)

9. Suggest deleting the jargon, if any.

10. Does it come to an adequate conclusion? If not, does more research need to be done?

APPENDIX E
COMMONLY USED EDITORIAL MARKS

Mark	Meaning
℘	Delete
#	Insert space
¶	Begin paragraph
no ¶	No paragraph, run in
∧	Caret (for inserting words, phrases, or punctuation)
tr	Transpose (tr)
⌣	Close space
℘	Delete, close space
|=|	Hyphen
⊤	Dash ("em dash")
ⓢⓟ	Spell out, change from numerical to word
ital	Italics (underline)
caps	Capital (caps)
sc	Small caps (sc)
lc	Lower case (lc)

stet	Stet (leave as is)
⊓	Move up
⊔	Move down
⊏	Move left
⊐	Move right
‖	Align

APPENDIX F

MAJOR HEALTH PROFESSION
BOOK PUBLISHERS

Robert J. Brady Co.
Division of Prentice-Hall
Bowie, Maryland 20715

John Wiley & Sons
605 Third Avenue
New York, New York 10016

Williams and Wilkins Co.
428 E. Preston Street
Balitmore, Maryland 21202

Harper & Row, Publishers
10 East 53rd Street
New York, New York 10022

Appleton-Century-Crofts
Division of Prentice-Hall
292 Madison Avenue
New York, New York 10017

C.V. Mosby Co.
118 Westline Industrial Drive
St. Louis, Missouri 63141

McGraw-Hill Book Co.
1221 Avenue of Americas
New York, New York 10020

136

W.B. Saunders
Division of CBS, Inc.
West Washington Square
Philadelphia, Pennsylvania 19105

Springer Publishing Co., Inc.
200 Park Avenue South
New York, New York 10003

APPENDIX G
SAMPLE RESUME

GEORGE O. SMITH, M.D.
  Chief of Surgery, Smith Clinic
  Professor of Surgery, Eastern University

HOME ADDRESS:	PHONE:
514 Golf Haven Dr.	GE 7-0436
Eastern, Pa.	

OFFICE ADDRESS:	PHONE:
31-103 The Boulevard	AD 3-4310
Eastern, Pa.	

POSITIONS HELD:
  Surgical Resident, The New York Hospital — 1961-63
  Orthopedic Surgical Resident, U. of Penn. Hospital —
    1963-65
  Private Practice — 1965-70
  Assistant Chief, Orthopedic Surgery, Eastern University
    1970-74
  Chief of Surgery, Eastern University — 1974-Present
  Associate Professor, Orthopedic Surgery, Eastern
    University — 1970-74
  Professor of Surgery, Eastern University —
    1974-Present

HONORS:
  Program Chairman, Orthopedic Surgery, American
    Medical Association 1977-Present

137

President — Eastern County Medical Society 1974-76
Board Certification, Orthopedic Surgery — 1972
Consultant in Orthopedic Surgery, Veterans
   Administration
Chairman, President's Committee on Orthopedic
   Combat Wounds — 1974-Present
Consultant in Orthopedic Surgery, University of
   Pennsylvania Hospital — 1972-Present
Editorial Consultant, *Journal of Orthopedic Surgery* —
   1974-Present

EDUCATION:
   B.S. — University of Wisconsin — 1956
   M.D. — Northwestern University, Cleveland — 1960

SOCIETIES (Member):
   Eastern (Pa.) County Medical Society
   American Medical Association
   American Academy of Orthopedic Surgeons
   National Academy of Sciences
   Industrial Surgeons Society
   Drug Information Association
   American Rehabilitation Society

PUBLICATIONS:
   Smith, George O., and Keel, John. *An Orthopedic
      Surgery Manual for Residents.* Prentice-Hall, Inc.,
      Englewood Cliffs, N. J., 1974. P. 108.
   Smith, George O. "Management of War-Induced Knee
      Injuries." Am. J. Orth. Surg. 3:34. March 1973.
      P. 1034-37.

BIBLIOGRAPHY — PART ONE

Barzun, J.: Simple and Direct: A Rhetoric for Writers, New York, Harper and Row, 1975.

Bernstein, T.M.: The Careful Writer, New York, Atheneum, 1975.

Dorland's Illustrated Medical Dictionary, 25th ed., Philadelphia, W.B. Saunders Co., 1974.

Elbow, P.: Writing Without Teachers, New York, Oxford University Press, 1976.

Hall, D.: Writing Well, 3rd ed., Boston, Little, Brown and Company,1979.

Hutchins, E.N.: Writing to be Read, Englewood Cliffs, NJ, Prentice-Hall, Inc., 1969.

Jacobs, H.B.: Writing and Selling Non-Fiction, Cincinnati, OH, Writer's Digest, 1967.

Newman, E.: Strictly Speaking, New York, Warner Books, 1975.

Nicholson, M.: A Practical Style Guide for Authors and Editors, New York, Holt, Rinehart and Winston, 1970.

Physicians' Desk Reference, 35th ed., Oradell, NJ, Medical Economics Co., 1981.

Strunk, W., Jr., White, E.B.: The Elements of Style, 3rd ed., New York, MacMillan Co., 1979.

White, V.P.: Grants: How to Find Out About Them and What to Do Next, New York, Plenum Publishing Co., 1975.

Zinsser, W.: On Writing Well: An Informal Guide for Writing, New York, Harper and Row, 1970.

Some Journals for Health Professionals

Nursing

American Journal of Nursing, 555 W. 57th St., New York 10019.

AORN Journal, 10170 E. Mississippi Ave., Denver, CO 80231.

Communicating Nursing Research, WICHE, Boulder, CO 80302.

Heart and Lung, The C.V. Mosby Co., 11830 Westline Ind. Dr., St. Louis, MO 63141.

Hospitals, JAHA, 840 N. Lake Shore Dr., Chicago, IL 60611.

Imprint, National Student Nurses Association, 10 Columbus Circle, New York 10019.

Journal of Continuing Education in Nursing, Journal of Gerontological Nursing, Journal of Nursing Education, and Occupational Health Nursing, 6900 Grove Road, Thorofare, NJ 08086.

Journal of Emergency Nursing, 3800 Capital City Blvd., Lansing MI 48906.

Journal of Nursing Administration and Nurse Educator, 12 Lakeside Park, 607 North Ave., Wakefield, MA 01880.

Journal of Nursing Midwifery, American College of Nurse Midwives, 1012 14th St., NW, Suite 801, Washington, DC 20005.

Journal of Obstetric, Gynecologic and Neonatal Nursing, 2350 Virginia Ave., Hagerstown, MD 21740.

Maternal Child Nursing, American Journal of Nursing Co., 555 W. 57th St., New York 10019.

Nursing '81, 132 Welsh Road, Horsham PA 19044.

Nursing Forum and Perspectives in Psychiatric Nursing, Box 218, Hillsdale, NJ 07642.

Nursing Outlook, 55 W. 57th St., New York, 10019.

Nursing Research, American Journal of Nursing Co., 555 W. 57th St., New York 10019.

Pediatric Nursing, N. Woodbury Road, Box 56, Pitman, NJ 08071.

Research in Nursing and Health, John Wiley & Sons, Inc., 605 3rd Ave., New York 10016.

RN Magazine, Kinderkamack Road, Oradell, NJ 07949.

Supervisor Nurse, 8 S. Michigan Ave., Chicago, IL 60603.

Western Journal of Nursing Research, Phillips-Allen, 1330 So. State College Blvd., Anaheim, CA 92806.

Psychology

American Psychologists, APA Monitor, Contemporary Psychology, Developmental Psychology, Journal of Abnormal Psychology, Journal of Consulting and Clinical Psychology, Psychological Bulletin, and Psychological Review, American Psychological Association, 1200 17th St., NW, Washington, DC 20036.

Behavior Today, Communications/Research/Machines, Inc., 317 14th St., Del Mar, CA 92014.

Human Behavior, Manson Western Corp., 12031 Wilshire Blvd., Los Angeles, CA 90025.

Practical Psychology for Physicians, Harcourt Brace Jovanovich, Inc., 757 Third Ave., New York 10017.

Pyschology Today, PO Box 2990, Boulder, CO 80302.

Social Work

Abstracts for Social Workers, National Association of Social Workers, 49 Sheridan Ave., Albany, NY 12210.

Channels, National Communications Council for Human Services, Inc., 815 Second Ave., New York 10017.

Children Today, Dept. of Health and Human Resources, Children's Bureau, PO Box 1182, Washington, DC

Clinical Social Work Journal, Human Sciences Press, 72 Fifth Ave., New York 10011.

Journal of Education for Social Work, Council on Social Work Education, 345 E. 46th St., New York 10017.

Journal of Marriage and Family Counseling, American Association of Marriage and Family Counselors, 225 Yale Ave., Claremont, CA 91711.

NASW News, National Association of Social Workers, Publication Sales Office, 49 Sheridan Ave., Albany, NY 12210.

Social Casework, Family Service Association of America, 44 E. 23rd St., New York 10010.

Social Work, National Association of Social Workers, 425 H St., NW, Washington, DC 20005.

Medicine

American Family Physician, American Academy of Family Physicians, 1740 W. 92nd St., Kansas City, MO 64114.

American Journal of Medicine, Donnelly Publishing Corp., 666 5th Ave., New York 10019.

Archives of General Psychiatry and Archives of Internal Medicine, American Medical Association, 535 N. Dearborn St., Chicago, IL 60610.

Hospitals, Journal of the American Hospital Association, 840 N. Lake Shore Dr., Chicago, IL 60611.

Lancet, Little, Brown and Co., 34 Beacon St., Boston, MA 02106.

New England Journal of Medicine, Massachusetts Medical Society, 10 Shattuck St., Boston, MA 02115.

BIBLIOGRAPHY — PART TWO
Writing the Research Report

Archer, JD: Attributes of a rejected manuscript, JAMA April 14, 1975.

Carnegie, ME: Rejection can be a challenge! Nursing Research, May-June, 1976.

Kratz C: How to write for publication: preparing a research article, Nursing Times, October 5, 1978.

Publication Manual of the American Psychological Association, 2nd ed., 1974, American Psychological Association, Washington, DC.

Soffer A. et al: Editorials, review articles, and case reports, Heart and Lung, March-April 1975.

Style Manual of the American Physical Therapy Association, 4th ed., 1976, American Physical Therapy Association, 1156 15th St., NW, Washington, DC 20005.

Styles MM: Why publish? Image, June, 1978.

Taylor SD: How to prepare an abstract, Nursing Outlook, September, 1967.

Witt P: Research writing tips, Physical Therapy, January, 1980.

Witt P: Research writing tips, introduction section and hypothesis, Physical Therapy, February 1980.

Witt P: Research writing tips: literature review, Physical Therapy, April 1980.

Witt P: Research writing tips: methods section, Physical Therapy, June, 1980.

Witt P: Research writing tips: results, Physical Therapy, July, 1980.

Witt P: Research writing tips: discussion, conclusion, references section, Physical Therapy, August, 1980.

Writing the Research Grant Proposal

Bloch D, Gortner SR, Sturdivant LW: The nursing research grants program of the Division of Nursing, US Public Health Service, J Nurs Admin, March, 1978.

Brodsky J (ed.): The Proposal Writer's Swipe File II: 14 professionally written grant proposals — prototypes of approaches, styles, and structures, Taft Products, Inc., 1000 Vermont Ave., NW, Washington, DC, 1976.

Dermer J: How to Write Successful Foundations Presentations, Public Service Materials Center, 104 E. 40th St., New York 10016, 1972.

DeBakey L, Debakey S: The art of persuasion: logic and language in proposal writing, Grants Magazine, March, 1978.

Eaves GN: The research grant application: an exercise in scientific writing, Grants Magazine, March, 1978.

Gortner SR: Research grant applications: what they are not and should be, Nurs Res, July-August, 1971.

Hall M: Developing Skills in Project Writing, Continuing Education Publications, 1633 SW Park, Portland, OR.

Jacquette FL, Jacquette BI: What Makes a Good Proposal, The Foundation Center, 888 7th Ave., New York, 1973.

Kiritz NJ: Program planning and proposal writing, The Grantmanship Center News, 1(3): 1-8, 1974. (reprint)

Kiritz NJ: Program planning and proposal writing, The Grantmanship Center News, May-June, 1979.

Kiritz NJ: Proposal checklist and evaluation form, The Grantmanship Center News, July-August, 1979.

Krathwohl DR: How to Prepare a Research Proposal, Syracuse Univ. Book Store, 303 University Place, Syracuse, NY, 1966.

Malasanos LJ: What is a proposal? What are its component parts? Is it an effective instrument in assessing funding potential of research ideas?, Nurs Res, May-June, 1976.

Masterman LE: The Mechanics of Writing Successful Federal Grant Applications, St. Louis, MO, Institute of Psychiatry, U. of Missouri School of Medicine, 1973.

Mayer RA: What Will a Foundation Look for When You Submit a Grant Proposal?, The Foundation Center, 888 7th Ave., New York, 1972.

National Health Council, Inc.: An Introduction to Grants and Contracts in Major HEW Health Agencies with annotated references, 2nd ed, Gov't Relations Handbook Series, No. 5, 1978, The Council, 70 W. 40th St., New York 10018.

Notter LE: Research grant applications and nursing research, Nurs Res, July-August, 1971.

Phillips TP: What is the difference between a research grant and a research contract, and how is information obtained on the contract approach?, Nurs Res, Sept.-Oct., 1975.

US Dept. of Health, Education and Welfare: Public Health Service, DHEW Publication No. (OS) 76-50,000, 1974, Grants Policy Statement, Washington, DC, Gov't. Printing Office.

White VP: Grants, How to Find Out About Them and What to Do Next, New York, Plenum Press, 1975.

INDEX